IN PURSUIT OF

Y · O · U · T · H

Everyday Nutrition for
Everyone Over 35

Betty Kamen and Si Kamen

DODD, MEAD & COMPANY   New York

Published by Dodd, Mead & Company, Inc.
79 Madison Avenue, New York, N.Y. 10016

Distributed in Canada by McClelland and Stewart Limited, Toronto

Manufactured in the United States of America

Designed by Joan Greenfield

First Edition

Library of Congress Cataloging in Publication Data

Kamen, Betty.
    In pursuit of youth.

    Bibliography: p. 215
    Includes index.
    1. Longevity—Nutritional aspects. 2. Aging—Nutri-
tional aspects. 3. Nutrition. I. Kamen, Si. II. Title.
QP85.K36   1984   613.2   83-27497
ISBN 0-396-08364-1

DISCLAIMER

All of the facts in this book have been very carefully researched, and have been drawn from the most prestigious medical journals. However, in no way are any of the suggestions meant to take the place of advice given by your doctor.

Every incident in this book is a real life story, experienced by friends, relatives, or by us personally, or reported in medical journals. Names have been changed to protect the chocolate freaks, the sugarholics, the cola addicts, the closet health nuts, and above all the innocent, who are doing as well as they know how, but simply do not know how—well enough.

to
ANTHONY GOLDMARK
whose life sparked our youth
and made us glad we feel so young!

CONTENTS

Foreword   vii

Acknowledgments   ix

Introduction   xi

Prologue   xiii

CHAPTER 1: The Exercise Connection   1

CHAPTER 2: Image Projection   28

CHAPTER 3: The Scale Association   71

CHAPTER 4: Food Consequences   106

CHAPTER 5: The Stress Effect   158

CHAPTER 6: Specifics for the Pursuit of Youth   177

CHAPTER 7: Immunity and the Pursuit of Youth   197

Appendix   215

References   218

Index   247

FOREWORD

By Abram Hoffer, M.D., Ph.D.
Fellow, Academy of Orthomolecular Psychiatry

Death and life are two sides of the same coin. One is impossible without the other. All living beings, from the simplest microorganism to the most complex human, must recycle organic molecules out of which life is constructed. There will never be eternal life for any individual.

Life's strongest imperative is survival—of the individual and of the species. Reproduction must precede death. Living organisms approach the end of their lives in different ways: by splitting (cell division); by disease or accident; or by becoming someone else's food supply. For most animal species life terminates rather abruptly, except for species such as man who have reached the top of the food chain. No animal species use man as their food.

During evolution our ancestors lived brief, very hectic lives. Predators and prey were locked into a never-ending fight for survival, each depending upon skills designed to ensure species survival. Survival genes are transmitted from individuals best able to survive in that particular niche. Any survival advantage which accrues after the reproductive period is over will not be of any genetic advantage. There will be a social advantage to species which maintain a social group.

As life-span expanded, the optimum productive period and death diverged more and more. But since fitness is transmitted at an age earlier than death, there has been no incentive to improve our genes beyond the reproductive age. If we had our optimum reproductive period at age eighty, we might have much superior human beings.

The problem is: can we improve our physiology so that we remain healthy as we age until we die? Nature requires a long time to solve these types of problems, but there is no reason we cannot use our intelligence and the information we have to hasten this process.

One of the fundamental changes occurred when life, which was anaerobic, became aerobic, i.e., required oxygen for the conversion of food to energy. But this created a new problem. Oxygen has a great affinity for organic matter. This is why a cut potato or apple turns brown. How does nature prevent this from happening in our body? Why do our lungs not oxidize? One solution is to have available molecules which prevent oxygen from combining. These are called antioxidants. In animals these are substances such as vitamin C, which is one of the water soluble antioxidants, and vitamin E, which is a fat soluble antioxidant. Most of the known antioxidants are derived from our food, if it is whole, fresh, and free of additives which increase the rate of oxidation.

Several theories explaining aging are being examined. My favorite is the free radical theory, i.e., that premature aging is due to an accumulation of free radicals. These are very reactive oxidizing molecules which may or may not contain oxygen. These free radicals age our tissues. Any factor which increases the free radical content will accelerate aging. These include too much oxygen, ozone, excessive sun, radiation, oxidizing additives, and a deficiency of antioxidants such as vitamin C, vitamin E, selenium, glutathione, some sulphydril polypeptides, and so on.

Any program designed to keep us healthy during a phase of our life which has not been genetically programmed for healthy longevity, must reverse all these deleterious factors. These will be some of the measures described in this valuable book.

ACKNOWLEDGMENTS

Montaigne said, "I quote others only the better to express myself." We are indebted to those whose words have aided the execution of our message.

Generally, we thank:

The caring, sharing medical profession for contributions to scientific journals which supplied much of the background for this book. Because it would have broken the narrative flow, we have not always given credit directly in the text for words, thoughts, and research. We have, however, cited every name in our references. The narrative approach was taken in an effort to translate important and life-enhancing medical information for the lay public.

Specifically, we thank:

Perle Kinney, for having gone untold extra miles (with unsurpassed genius) out of sheer devotion as a true friend;

Serafina Corsello, M.D., whose dazzling intellect and perspicacity provided a major contribution to Chapter 5, to our work, and to our lives in general;

Kathi and Joe Goldmark, for rounding up people worldwide—contributing cultural insights in the pursuit of youth;

Joseph Consentino, M.D., for wisdom on image projection—a major contribution to Chapter 2;

Michael Kamen, for an understanding of human nature that makes all behavior so clear—adding to our personal cognition and tolerance of everyone we know;

Yury Agureyev, for his talent, humor, and willingness to help, always with enthusiasm;

Warren Levin, M.D., who contributed details on the complexities of fatty acid metabolism and nutrient supplementation, and, through his daring to break from tradition, has given new life to thousands of patients (even though his mother doesn't think he's a "real" doctor);

Howard Bezoza, M.D., for permitting us to pick his brains in the middle of his busy day;

Abram Hoffer, M.D., for his pioneering work and the eloquent foreword of this book;

Jeffrey Bland, Ph.D., for burning midnight oil to update concepts and research on the frontier of medical nutrition;

Marshall Mandell, M.D., for sharing his unique clinical research on allergic symptoms;

Rob Benowicz, for tedious studies on drugs and drug interactions—contributing to the credibility of our statements;

Diana Dalton, M.A., for sharing her extensive investigation and clinical experience on the nutritional management of menopause and menstrual difficulties;

William Oliver, M.D., for impressive, mind-boggling journeys to distant and primitive cultures—which brought us the "salt talks."

Helen E. Fisher, Ph.D., for fascinating anthropology wisdom;

Bill Holub, Ph.D., for a rare holistic approach to the biochemistry of the human organism;

Charles Stroebel, M.D.; John Douglass, M.D.; and Elliott Goldwag, M.D. for their innovative interpretations of scientific facts;

Dan Nidess, for providing the vehicle through which books like this get into the hands of people who benefit from them;

And finally, two people whose contributions are unparalleled: Carlton Fredericks, Ph.D., for making it all happen long ago; and Evan Marshall, editor and agent, for making it all happen today.

INTRODUCTION

Midnight is a late hour.
The print in the telephone book is not as dark as it used to be.
"Get up and go" has gone.
There are two nightly trips to the bathroom.
Someone has told you to pull in your stomach, but you already did.

These are the realities for anyone who is approaching (or has already rounded) the turning point. Are these events inevitable? Are they normal, or merely average? Can you hold them at bay? Can you reverse them?

When did you get entangled in these aging parameters anyway? Could it have been all those violations over the years? The coffee? The cigarettes? Those cocktail parties? What about heredity? Not to worry. Grandpa lived to be 94. But Aunt Molly died at 56!

The facts? Aging doesn't happen just like that. No one ever ages instantly. It's a state arrived at slowly—the consequence of a complexity of happenings. The outward presentation of aging represents the balance scale overloaded: on one side, natural forces are working to keep your machinery in good working order; on the other, contaminants, indiscretions, and the ticking clock are working *against* that order. But again, the over-tax is a slow process, and it can be delayed.

In Pursuit of Youth introduces specific positive measures to optimize life quality at any age. This is done with a minimum of restrictions because we are, after all, real people. We suggest easy guidelines for reversing the aging process.

No particular theory of nutrition is evangelized. But there is background information—correlating the relationship between "corruptions" (both personal and imposed) and the wearing down of your body—which allows you to put these facts into context. Nutrition, exercise, and other life-style facets have a role to play in the genesis of aging, and thereby in the pursuit of youth.

★   ★   ★

Prayer indeed is good, but while calling on the gods, a man should himself lend a hand.

—Hippocrates, *Regimen*

PROLOGUE

At age twenty-five, most of the organs of your body have a higher functional capacity than is usually necessary. This is called *organ reserve*. The aging process reduces organ reserve. Some organs lose their reserve more quickly than others. Some people lose organ reserve more quickly than others.

Why are we robbed of this reserve? Is it genetics? Environment? Both? Why does a young person have less body fat, more blood volume, and more lean body mass than his or her parents? We know these changes are *average*. But are they *normal?* "Average" is that which is typical; that which conforms to the common. "Normal" is that which is natural; that which conforms to nature.

When you have reached the point at which symptoms appear, there is no more reserve. You have reached the turning point. This is sickness after youth. You can now feel and see the process which literally started years before.

The causes for organ reserve loss have been theorized since time began. Among old wives' tales of medical folklore there are true elixirs of youth, and also dead ends. No clue has ever gone unnoticed or untried. Included in the potpourri of proclamations are sex (with theories wavering between total abstinence and extreme licentiousness), color, herbs, adversity, soured milk, spring water, mercury compounds, magic, meditation, and brews prepared from substances as esoteric as snakeskin and as mundane as mixtures of garden variety vegetables.

New-age youth precepts are here, along with new-age health mastery. They go hand in hand: new medical modalities can keep you healthier, with youth and pleasure a fringe benefit—a magnificent gift. We have made an extensive study of all the proposals—those of yesteryear, and those hot off today's computer terminals. When the final answer is in, it is more than likely that we'll learn that aging is complex, that it is the result of an interplay of relationships, a kaleidoscope of processes. (One can envision a twenty-first century snake oil pitch person on a soap box, shouting, "step right up and get your deoxyribonucleic acid. Maximal synaptic formation guaranteed.")

But that's tomorrow. Here's a compendium of foods and factors that delay or accelerate the aging process according to theories old and current:

☆POSITIVES☆

Activity	Liver
B complex	Low animal fat
Calcium	Low-calorie diets
Complex carbohydrates	Meditation
Cultured milk	Nutrient dense foods
DNA	Quality protein
Eggs	RNA
Enhanced immune system	Root plants
Enzymes	Sex
Fish	Sprouts
Garden variety vegetables	Trace elements
Herbs	Vitamin A
Homeostasis	Vitamin C
Leafy vegetables	Vitamin E
Leanness	Water
Legumes	Yeast

▫NEGATIVES▫

Additives
Alcohol
Caffeine
Drugs

Excessive sun
Food processing (canning; freezing; storing)
Infection
Obesity
Pollution
Rancid fat (potential sources: french fries;
    salad dressings; processed oils;
    potato chips; anything deep-fried)
Retirement
Stress
Tobacco

☆**Positive**☆ and ▢**negative**▢ longevity factors have been summarized. Wherever a ☆**positive**☆ is mentioned, it appears this way: ☆**Vitamin C**☆. Wherever a ▢**negative**▢ is indicated, it appears this way: ▢**french fries**▢.

A few ☆**positives**☆ and ▢**negatives**▢ not listed specifically in the compendium have been "flagged" in the text because they are components of the ☆**plus**☆ or ▢**minus**▢ aging factors cited.

Although more and more people are living to advanced ages, a huge proportion suffers from chronic disease *with the incidence of such disease increasing yearly.* Forestalling the consequences of a sick old age is the key to pursuit of youth.

If a more healthful life-style delays aging—and the evidence points in that direction—let's get on with it. For those of you who remember when bank robbers pulled up to a bank and got a parking space, it's not too late. The aging process can be slowed down and sometimes even reversed. For those of you who don't remember when the small voice within you was conscience instead of a transistor radio, how lucky you are. You can't help getting older, but you don't have to get old.

★   ★   ★

"To know how to grow old is the master work of wisdom, and one of the most difficult chapters in the great art of living."
                            —Henri Frédéric Amiel, 1800s

CHAPTER 1

The Exercise Connection

A man confided to a friend: "I'm almost sixty-five years old, but I look younger because I have worked out at the gym for years and years. I have saved half a million, and have fallen madly in love with a dashing young blonde of nineteen. Do you think I'd have a better chance to have her marry me if I told her I'm only fifty?"

"I think you'd have a better chance to land her," answered his friend, "if you told her you're eighty."

The Track

They are all going in the same direction, covering miles, but not distance. Strangers pass each other and say, "Good morning." No one is excluded because of age: no one is too young or too old. Nor are there species restrictions: the canine contingent is in attendance, one or two dogs maintaining a rather loose proximity to their masters. It is the only place where shoe styles are identical and sweaty brows acceptable. Although under □stress□, the participants are not only calm, but euphoric. Local residents come to the track at the high school to stretch or to walk or to run.

But don't get the wrong impression about the sociality of it all. Although it may be the friendliest group of strangers in town, we live in an era of depersonalization. Few and far between are front porches (those that do exist are rarely occupied), neighborhood grocery stores,

1

or strollers stopping to chat. As the numbers of people in the world increase, we are becoming more anonymous. This is reflected at the high school track where there are polite "hellos," rare personal exchanges, and frequent comments about the weather and exercising conditions. Everyone is as generic as unbranded cans of vegetables on supermarket shelves. The identities are "Young Man with Head Set," "Old Gray-Haired Guy," "Large-Bosomed Lady in T-Shirt," "The Couple," and so on. There are no coffee-klatch relationships.

The commonality of the group is the hour of the day set aside for each individual to:

1. deliver more oxygen to muscles
2. allow lungs to get rid of more carbon dioxide
3. increase tiny blood vessels throughout body cells
4. make those same blood vessels more flexible
5. increase bowel function efficiency
6. encourage better sleeping habits
7. experience less fatigue
8. lower blood pressure
9. improve glucose tolerance for better sugar metabolism
10. strengthen hearts
11. lower concentrations of "bad-guy" low-density lipoproteins, while increasing concentrations of "good-guy" high-density lipoproteins (both are components of the cholesterol control system of the body)
12. lower triglyceride levels
13. release the brain's natural morphine-like compounds known as endorphins
14. stimulate lymph systems

In summary, they are enjoying what may be a significant aging "antibiotic": aerobics.

All this they share as their bodies journey the track day after day after day. "Hi." "Muddy today." "Damn rain again." "Gorgeous day."

The group of strangers breathes deeply and no one accuses them of being obscene.

AEROBNIC #1

Running Risks

Bob Smith is a physician and ex-jogger. His metamorphosis from running to walking occurred because the good doctor witnessed too many running casualties. Medical journal surveys indicate that 35 percent of runners who cover sixty miles or more each week develop knee, foot, ankle, shin, back, or other musculoskeletal injuries within a year's time. Bone loss, similar to postmenopausal skeletal loss, occurs in young women who exercise excessively.[1] Other injuries may be incurred by dog bites, ▫sunburn▫, and motor vehicle accidents.

Although a large percentage of smokers quit ▫smoking▫ after beginning a program of running (81 percent of men and 75 percent of women), and many lose more than ten pounds,[2] Doctor Smith believes these same goals can be achieved with less trauma via ☆*fast walking*☆—unless you have been running from early on, and are following an exemplary life-style in other dimensions as well.

Among Bob Smith's own patients, he reports the following:

Patient A: Ran with arms acutely flexed at elbows, which compressed the radial nerve, resulting in numbness and tingling in left arm. Patient advised to run with arms less flexed, which patient found difficult to do. When patient stopped running and started walking briskly, patient's arms swung freely, and with ease. All symptoms disappeared.[3]

Patient B: Experienced blurring in eye after running ten miles. Dehydration and tissue damage may have contributed to patient's vascular occlusion (closing off of blood vessels). Recommendation: start exercise from scratch, *slowly* building up—and walk, do not run. Inadequate training could precipitate such symptoms.[4] Exercise regularly, progressing *gradually* to increased distance and speed.

Patient C: Well known to women who jog—condition of simple irritation of nipples caused by friction against shirt. Happens to women who do not wear bra while jogging. Situation remedied with coat of vaseline or talcum powder, or wearing blouse made of smooth hard silk rather than usual T-shirt, or *walking* instead of running, all of which reduce friction. Needless to say "joggers' nipples" are self-healing if further trauma avoided. Long-distance male runners are also familiar with problem, preventing pain and bleeding with tape.[5] (Hope it isn't too painful when tape is removed from hairy chest.)

Patient D: Bloody urine was complaint, result of repeated impact of empty bladder against prostate. Patient advised not to empty bladder before running, or to reduce impact by replacing running with *fast walking.* (Women protected from problem because of different anatomy.)[6]

Patient E: Suffered bronchial attacks when running in cold weather. Hard outdoor exercise in low temperature impinges cool, dry air on tracheal and bronchial mucosa. Mucus thickened, movements of tracheal cilia slowed, and tracheal nerve endings stimulated, causing bronchial spasms.[7] Recommendations: don't work so hard at exercising (walk, don't run), or wear jogger's mask which allows warm, moist air to be inspired from within patient's own track suit.[8]

Patient F: No menstruation for over a year; concerned because of interest in becoming pregnant. Jogging can reduce proportion of body fat and lead to reduction in circulating hormones necessary for fertility. Over 50 percent of women who run sixty miles a week are amenorrheic. Women often experience amenorrhea when body fat rapidly falls below 10 percent. (The average well-nourished young woman has 20 to 25 percent fat content.[9]) Ovulation and conception achieved within eight weeks of cessation of jogging.[10] Patient encouraged to continue walking during pregnancy because of recent reports of easier deliveries for properly exercised mothers-to-be.

Then there are the patients with foot, leg, and knee breakdowns. Tendinitis, hamstring pull, bursitis of the greater trochanter (part of the upper femur), forearm extensor overload, shinsplints (strain of long muscles that control the toes; pain along shin bone), and plantar (sole of the foot) pain, among them. Dr. Smith's patients prefer the diagnosis of jogger's foot, jogger's heel, jogger's ankle, jogger's leg, jogger's knee, jogger's thigh, jogger's hip,[11] rather than nomenclature which defines the specifics of anatomy malfunctions.

Of those who run regularly to an endurance level, 60 percent suffer chronic lower extremity injuries.[12] In a study of 120 middle-aged joggers, 240 injuries surfaced![13] Of course walking is not entirely without its hazards. Bob himself was a victim recently—an episode he chooses not to broadcast: he suffered frostbite of the penis. Upon returning from his walk one cold morning, he ached: glans frigid, red, tender upon manipulation and anesthetic to light touch. Immediate therapy involved removing his polyester double-knit trousers and Dacron-cotton undershorts. Response was rapid and complete after rewarming. (His wife arrived on the scene in time to help with the therapy.) Bob diagnosed the pathogenesis as tissue response to high air velocity at below-zero temperature, penetrating the interstices of polyester and continuing through anterior opening of undershorts. He now wears athletic supporter and old, tight, cotton warm-up pants. (No recurrences are expected.) [14]

Among other frequent metabolic imbalances caused by running, is the problem of hemoglobinuria (hemoglobin in the urine) and hemoglobinemia (anemia). Hemoglobin is the oxygen-carrying pigment of the blood. A condition called "march hemoglobinuria" was identified in the nineteenth century when soldiers marched for long periods of time. It is believed that twentieth-century runners and joggers often suffer march hemoglobinuria and do not know it. Today's exercising anemia is ascribed to iron deficiency, since iron is lost through hemoglobinuria. Because many runners have hemoglobinemia after running only two to six miles, and virtually all marathon runners are affected, Dr. Smith encourages die-hard runners to take these precautions:

wear shoes with resilient insoles
apply a thin layer of vaseline or similar lubricant on the soles of
    feet before running
avoid heavy, stamping strides
avoid hard roads in favor of grass or dirt
avoid hills
avoid extremes of weather
avoid racing against fellow joggers or the clock
avoid running after eating
avoid running if not feeling up to par
stop jogging *before* you feel you cannot take another step
wear a hat on any sunny day

Dr. Smith offers a clear description of what happens each time the runner's foot hits the pavement: shock waves are transmitted from the heel up through the ankle, leg, knee, thigh, hip, and back. The more extensive and vigorous the run, the more impacts received. [15] Bob can only present the information. He believes that ultimately each person is responsible for his or her own health, a rare attitude for a physician.

It has been one hundred years since the first reports of march hemoglobinuria first appeared in medical journals.[16] Will it take another hundred years before we fully understand the mechanisms? Another hundred years before all nonprofessional athletes are aware of precautions necessary to avoid its consequences?

Hemoglobinuria can also be induced by drumming, an exercise of great physical intensity. A very unusual research project was undertaken at the University of Pennsylvania hospital. A series of sessions on conga and bongo drums was initiated. The concerts became part of controlled, scientific data. With each successive concert, the hemoglobinuria problem experienced by the musicians was intensified. Drummers in the West Indies, where the drums are placed on absorbent earth, do not experience these difficulties. In America, of course, they are placed on hard floors.[17] It may be that paradigm again, thought Bob, when he read about this. Anything more natural may be more protecting—possibly even for the drummer.

Walking Works Wonders

Bob did not go directly from running to walking. An intermediate step was bicycling to his office every day. After a while he developed numbness in the fourth and fifth digits of each hand. When lack of feeling spread up his forearms, he related the problem to his backpack. He carried heavy books and papers in the pack, tightening the straps to keep the weight high on his back. He considered getting a bike rack, but decided that race-walking moved more of his body and, in general, was a better exercise discipline.[18] Raymond Dreyfack, a walking expert, says:

Walking uses muscles all over the body, and everything comes into play. You get the same cardiovascular benefit out of thirty minutes of brisk walking as you get from twenty minutes of running . . . London bus drivers had more coronary heart diseases than conductors who walked back and forth in the vehicles to take tickets.[19]

Dreyfack's example of the London conductors is one of many. Whether you compare railway switchmen with railway clerks, postal carriers with postal clerks, college athletes with their more sedentary classmates, or farmers and longshoremen with the rest of the community, the active members of each pair will have less clinical evidence of coronary heart disease.[20]

Bob enjoys reading an occasional article in his medical journals describing the Masai, a nomadic East African tribe, which uses jogging as a basic form of locomotion whether at work or at play. The Masai run, rather than walk, as they move through the day. Needless to say they have an incredible level of physical fitness. At the other end of the scale are the affluent groups (that's us) for whom the automobile and myriad labor-saving devices have virtually removed ☆**physical activity**☆ as a necessity of life and living. (Americans are the only people who don't even have to shake a bottle of milk. Milk is not homogenized any place else.) Lifelong physical activity should be stressed for future generations.

Bob Smith does not like to tell a patient categorically that he or she cannot run, unless it places the patient at obvious risk. He also knows that the average person is not fully knowledgeable concerning the detriments—if running has not been a lifetime endeavor. Tight straps, wrong fabrics, dehydration, weather factors, body breakdowns, systemic breakdowns—all can be □**stressors**□ when an exercise program is too long or too vigorous. It is true, of course, that more people die from inactivity than exercise, but there is a happy medium. If Bob had his way, everyone would start running at an early age, or walk briskly forevermore.

Bob's enthusiasm in imparting the importance of exercise sometimes gets patients so fired up that they overdo it. (If a little is good, more is better.) Equally frustrating are his efforts to get totally inactive patients to move—to blow balloons or move their toes up and down, if that's all they can do. He'll even recommend a rocker for the very resistant. The action used for putting the rocker into motion stretches leg muscles and also stimulates circulation.

Bob does not particularly like most clinical tests because they are not sophisticated enough to be completely accurate. He does, however, administer a few tests when he thinks it will serve the purpose of getting his point across. He knows no other way that graphically demonstrates to his patients just how their bodies are functioning, or malfunctioning, even though results may be misleading. He is mindful of the inconsistencies. For example, if someone is in good shape when on the treadmill, it will take a long time to get to maximum heart rate. But if the patient has certain kinds of heart disease, he or she won't reach that maximum either. In addition, some people run the risk of getting unwanted information on treadmill tests, which may be an advantage or disadvantage, depending on treatment prescribed. It is up to the patient to evaluate proposed medical intervention.

Aerobic exercise is beneficial for some emotional disorders. The phenomena of both euphoria and addiction suggest participation of the central nervous system in response to regular physical ☆activity☆.[21] Because of this, Bob expends much energy coaxing patients who are depressed and fatigued to enter regular exercise programs. However, the patients for whom it would be most beneficial are the most resistant and difficult to motivate.

An additional windfall of regular walking schedules stems from being outdoors. Exposing both body and eyes to daylight causes an increased output of various glandular secretions.[22] Bob does caution against exercising in traffic-congested areas. Tests show that carbon monoxide levels of city runners are comparable to those found in habitual □smokers□. Both the breathing rate and air intake are increased during forceful exertion, encouraging greater inhalation of this □**pollutant**□. Walking engenders less □**stress**□ of this kind.[23]

As Dr. Bob Smith scurries around the track (he is now clocking twelve-minute miles—not bad for a walker), he envisions a world in which everyone moves aerobically. He wishes his colleagues would not write any more articles about cholesterol, and would stop bothering about whether fats are saturated or unsaturated. Isn't there enough evidence which shows that the more habitual exercise anyone takes, the less likely one is to be troubled by coronary disease?[24] He notices "Old Gray-Haired Guy" has picked up steam, and even more exciting, he has picked up his posture.

AEROBNIC #2

Learning a New Word

"Aerobics" is a new word for Ben Carpenter. In his youth, he assumed that if he lived to be an octogenarian, he would know all there is to know. "I'm so old," he keeps telling people, "I remember when air was clean and sex was dirty, not the other way round. I remember when there were no deductions from a man's weekly pay until he brought it home. Why, they no longer sell parts for the typewriter my family bought for my *sixty-fifth* birthday. In fact," continues Ben with a twin-kle, "I'm so old that my first typewriter typed in pencil. But if they keep inventing new words and new ways, my vocabulary and experi-ences will continue to increase along with the lines on my face."

Ben's interest in etymology sent him to the dictionary, and he learned that aerobic means able to live, grow, or take place only where free oxygen is present. His grandson explained that aerobic exercises are those which make the heart accelerate for a sustained period of time, causing a need for more air (oxygen). Aerobic exercises are run-ning, fast walking, swimming, rope jumping, biking—any kind of ☆ac-tivity☆ that is not stop-and-start, but go-go-go. "What counts," ex-plained his grandson, "is that the exercise is kept up for a period of time and that it is practiced daily or at least five times a week. The object is to improve those organs and systems involved in the body's processing of oxygen—the heart, lungs, and blood vessels. As the heart is strengthened, its work load is lightened."

Ben, at 83, wanted all the help he could get. If aerobics lightened the load, aerobics he would try. Not that Ben had ever been seden-tary—he just never allowed himself the luxury of a purposeful exercise regimen, a planned activity. "In the good old days," said Ben, "when a man finished his day's work, he needed rest; nowadays he needs ex-ercise. But then, in the good old days we used to speak of the good old days."

For years Ben had been saying you can tell how healthy a man is by what he takes two at a time—stairs or pills. Many of his friends had already self-destructed. He found himself quoting his father: "If youth only knew; if age only could." Well, the world is full of sur-prises. He was learning from youth, and the message was that if aging is inevitable, its pace might be retarded with (that funny word) aero-bics. He heard a young fellow of 65 proudly announce, after an aero-bics event, "winning at my age is an accomplishment." Ben thought, "*Getting* to my age is an accomplishment! But I'll try it—this aero-bics."

Benefits at Any Age

Armed with his definitions, Ben went to the library to do some research before embarking on "this aerobics." He learned from a book by Dr. Jeffrey Bland that:

The conditioning effect occurs when your body recognizes that you are asking things of it which it had long ago forgotten about. As you force the cells of your body to produce energy during aerobic exercise, the tiny subcellular sites of energy production are encouraged to become more efficient and also actually to increase in number. These sites of energy production within all cells are called *mitochondria.* . . . Aerobic exercise "tunes up" mitochondrial function.[25]

Ben also learned that his body would increase its ability to deliver ☆**nutrients**☆, that he would increase the capacity of his lungs, and that he would enlarge major blood vessels. These advantages would only accompany the aerobics. He read that the risk of developing coronary heart disease in men reporting regular, forceful exercise was about a third of that in comparable men not exercising aerobically. The protective effect continues throughout middle age.[26] Since Ben considered middle age anything from 35 to 110, he decided that aerobics was for him.

Ben dug up another bit of reinforcing information. Hypoxia is the diminished availability of oxygen to body tissues. He learned that hypoxia and aging cause similar declines in metabolism, such as decreased mental capacities.[27] If he could bring more oxygen to his tissues by exercising, he might forestall mental function decline. Death itself does not disturb him. Losing his "marbles" does!

Ben remembers when strict prohibition of exercise was the order of the day for high blood pressure. Now exercise is regular clinical prescription for that symptom. Pressure is lowered for four to ten hours after aerobics, possibly because it results in general vasodilation (a state of increased diameter of the blood vessels). The healthier the individual, the more rapid the return to normal, following exertion.[28]

Ben is determined to follow through. Dr. Paul Dudley White said, "Legs are our second heart. To stay healthy, a person must use his or her legs."[29] Ben believes that in exercise, as in good deeds, the reward must also lie in the act itself. Doctors reporting in the *New England Journal of Medicine* agree with Ben.[30]

Ben thoroughly researched one other aspect of aerobics: age. Was he too old to move his body aerobically? Could aerobics be harmful for someone who still has TV dinners in front of the radio? Was he buying oats for a dead horse? He learned that:

- The aging heart, nervous, and muscular systems respond well to aerobic training. The capacity and the ☆**enzyme**☆ function of an aged muscle increases with training to similar extents and by essentially the same mechanisms as those identified in young muscles. The percent of improvement with training is similar in all age groups.[31]

- Physically trained individuals appear to have postponed, at least partially, the physical ravages of age. They appear to be physiologically younger than untrained individuals.[32]
- When older people are tested for their responses to motor tasks, such as tapping time and simple reactions of hands and feet, their responses are related to survival: those who are slower than their age group (but biologically older) die at a younger age.[33] Fast walking, commencing at any age, improves psychomotor speed tasks such as those used in this test.
- The rate of adaptation to exercise slows as a person becomes older, and the recovery period following effort may be prolonged.[34] The advice is to increase time, but not intensity, and allow for longer cool-down periods.
- Investigating cardiorespiratory training in older people, it was found they had at least as great a response as younger subjects.[35,36,37]
- Fitness can be achieved with continuous vigorous walking for regular periods of time each day, no matter what age or level of activity one has participated in before starting.[38]
- The loss of bone ☆**calcium**☆ both from lack of use and age contributes to an increased propensity to fractures.[39] ☆**Exercised**☆ bones do not demineralize. They are far less likely to break or lose their range of motion.[40]
- Exercised lungs still exhibit changes of age, but are far less diminished in their capacity compared to the lungs of sedentary people.[41]
- Studies of the effects of exercise on people over age 60 show that with sufficiently severe regimens continued for ten to twelve weeks, there is an improvement in physical capacity. Subjects also report feeling better and attitudes are improved. Physical exercise can even sharpen cognitive decisional and memory functions.[42]
- Levels of human growth hormone do not change very much from childhood to old age. There is a beneficial increase of this hormone during exercise which occurs as much in an older person as in a young person.[43,44]

Four-Mile Crawl or Three-Mile Race?

A final caveat came from Ben's grandson: "Gramps, start slowly."

"I'm not sure I have time to start anything slowly."

"You will if you make aerobic walking a habit. And remember, although more calories are burned moving faster, the prolonged moderate rhythmic endurance of your walk is more important."

"Don't they teach you anything in physics these days? To move a given weight a mile requires just as much energy whether it is moved faster or more slowly. Maybe it takes me all night to do what I used to do all night, but I still remember that energy expended is a function of mass times distance, and time is not a factor in this equation. So how can I burn more calories walking faster?"

"That's true in a mechanical, mathematical concept, but your body is not a machine. If you run hard for six miles, you burn 20 percent more calories than you do walking the same distance. This has been proved in physiological studies. The closer you get to your maximum potential, the more energy you expend. For you, the distance you go is far more important than the speed at which you travel."[45]

Now that Ben has been walking aerobically for a few months, he feels that his entire body is operating more efficiently—the only machine in his experience that works better the *more* it is used. And it is so easy! The mechanics of walking are built in: as strides are taken, abdominal muscles contract to support their share of weight; deeper breathing is aided by the increased effort of the diaphragm and rib muscles; shoulder and neck muscles contribute as they help to hold the head erect.[46]

Ben had a hunch that if all the members of his senior citizens group walked with him, he would be attending more parties and fewer funerals. And as for that word "aerobics," Ben had been using it for years. Except he called it "moving hardy."

He greeted "Tall Young Man with Blue Cap," admiring the way he seemed to fly effortlessly as he circled the track. He wished he had known about all this sixty years ago. But even at 83, he reminds himself that today is still the first day of the rest of his life.

AEROBNIC #3

High Test Fuel For Runners

Mike Cannon is unmarried, mid-thirties. He is what his school coaches called "a natural athlete." Mike has been running every day for so many years that he can't really say how old he was when he started.

There is a family joke, often repeated when he and his brother and father discuss well-being. His brother says, "Smoke pot. You will enter a world where everything is blurred and fantastic." His father says, "I get the same result by misplacing my glasses." For Mike, running creates the high.

Noncompetitive, Mike is not interested in marathons. He runs no more than twenty or twenty-five miles a week. But he is concerned with deriving the best possible personal experience as he moves rapidly around the track. Therefore, Mike has made a study of foods and their effect on both his performance and health.

Glycogen is the chief carbohydrate storage material in animals. It is formed by and largely stored in the liver, and to a lesser extent in muscles. The first response to exercise is a depletion of glycogen from muscle. If exercise is continued long enough, fatty acids are then utilized.[47]

Glucose is the fuel that forms glycogen. Does that mean that glucose ingestion before or during exercise is the answer? Mike learned the hard way: no indeed! Glucose ingestion may prevent hypoglycemia (low blood sugar) during exercise, but it does not affect endurance or delay exhaustion.[48] However, an increase in glycogen *stores* will enhance endurance.[49] How then does one increase muscle glycogen stores?

Basic nutrition needs do not vary with activity. Nor, for that matter, do they vary for inactive people, but it should be noted that the effect of nutrient deficiency may be more deleterious for the athlete because of increased energy requirements.[50] Metabolic processes, however, work more efficiently for the exerciser than the sedentary because a larger percentage of food is properly digested and assimilated. The exerciser gets more nutrients from the same amount of food without a diet change. Nonetheless, people have been attempting to feed themselves "high test fuel" for optimal athletic performance for at least 2500 years. (Greek athletes had their theories too.) If you take inventory of ergogenic (work enhancing) dietary aids before a competition, you will note that people are consuming honey, sweet drinks, vitamins, gelatin, bee pollen, wheat germ oil, dextrose, protein supplements, even steaks—regardless of the sport involved.

How to Store Glycogen

Mike tried them all. As each sports magazine espoused one or another particular diet, he responded. At one time it was believed that protein builds muscles. We now know that as long as the minimum requirements of protein are met, the size of the muscle depends on the physical demands made upon it, and not on an oversupply of protein. Since most protein foods are high in fat, the high protein diet may also be a high fat diet. This is not advantageous for the exerciser. Gastric emptying of fat takes five hours as compared with two hours for bread or cereal. A full stomach is a great impediment to performance.[51]

The first articles extolling the virtues of the ☆complex carbohydrate☆ diet appeared in sports and nutrition journals. Mike was delighted when the information finally filtered up (down?) to the establishment tabloids:

- *American Journal of Clinical Nutrition:* Forty-eight hours after exercise the ☆complex carbohydrate☆ diet results in significantly higher muscle glycogen levels than a simple carbohydrate diet.[52]
- *Acta Physiologica Scandinavica:* The capacity to perform heavy exercise increases 300 to 400 percent when the preceding diet is changed from carbohydrate-poor to carbohydrate-rich [☆complex carbohydrates☆].[53]
- *Nutrition Today:* Endurance for prolonged aerobic work is maintained an average of four hours after several days on a high carbohydrate diet, three hours after a mixed diet, and only one hour after a diet high in fat. This increased vigor is thought to be due to the increased glycogen stored in muscles associated with high carbohydrate diets.[54]
- *American Heart Journal:* Aerobic activities are correlated positively with increases in high-density lipoproteins, which in turn are positively correlated with better heart health.[55]

Mike now understands that increased glycogen stores in muscles are associated with high ☆complex carbohydrate☆ diets.

An untrained athlete is more likely to have his endurance limited by glycogen since the novice consumes more glycogen at a higher rate.[56] Dr. Daniel Hanley, an expert on muscle function, explains:

Only when the muscle can be assured of an adequate supply of oxygen, glucose, and fatty acids does it have the fuel to run, and only after the brain selects what muscles should be used does the body have a direction in which to move. Without any one organ component, this machine works poorly, if at all. All the parts have the ability to adapt and become more efficient with practice. Just as the right kind of gas is necessary for the efficiency of your car, a trained muscle, if it has been fueled with too little or the wrong kind of nutrients, will not perform. In the end, it is the muscles that must do the task defined by the brain with fuel supplied to it by the heart, liver, and lungs.

Muscle tissue is like a gasoline engine: A full tank of gas doesn't help a small engine go faster than a large engine. The car with the larger fuel tank will travel for a longer time if it is compared to a car with the same engine size, but a smaller fuel tank.[57]

Mike remembers when his high school coach recommended downing a salt-rich drink after a perspiration provoking endeavor. If Coach Kelly only knew then what we know now! The sodium concentration found in sweat is lower than that found in blood or the fluid between the cells. Therefore, sodium concentration increases in your blood when sweat is secreted, no matter how much fluid is available to the athlete. A salt-rich drink plainly has no advantage relative to water at this stage.[58] A cumulative deficiency of sodium, however, is likely if heavy sweating continues for several days, if the diet is not replenishing sodium supplies. Potassium may also be lost in perspiration. A diet high in natural ☆complex carbohydrates☆ supplies all the sodium and potassium needed, in ratios necessary for optimal cell health. Among such foods: celery, bananas, raw carrots, avocados, and apricots. (Actually, fruits should not be classified as complex carbohydrates because of their simple sugar content.) ☆Eggs☆, although not a complex carbohydrate, contain an excellent sodium/potassium ratio.

An additional asset of the complex carbohydrate, or vegetarian meal, concerns ☆iron☆ absorption. If the meal has a high content of ☆ascorbic acid☆, there will be an extremely high rate of iron absorption. In fact, one study which shows only a threefold variation in iron content in meals tested, resulted in a *sevenfold* difference in iron absorption. Even though the foods with the highest iron content contained only three times the amount of iron as the low iron foods, the amount of iron absorbed was much greater because these foods also contained vitamin C. The meals with the low iron absorption were comprised of meat and fish, which contain very little vitamin C.[59] This is important because of the fact that iron levels are often compromised in those who exercise with might and main. *Vitamin C potentiates iron absorption.*

Mike runs on this particular school track every morning before work. He told many friends about "Old Gray-Haired Guy" who seems to be walking faster and faster every day. He has not told his friends about "Lovely Lady," with whom he exchanges smiles.

AEROBNIC #4

Ballet Is Not Enough

Meg Morgan barely touches the ground as she darts ahead. Her grace and posture are the culmination of years of dance training. Despite the early hour, this is Meg's second round of body maneuvers for the day. She has already spent sixty minutes on elongation exercises, front thigh shape-ups, bending, stretching, kicking, pulling, pushing. But here on the track she is moving aerobically.

Young as she is (mid-thirties), Meg is already an "old" dancer. It has been her observation that former athletes and ex-dancers often become far less active by the time they reach middle age, and are too often heavier than their contemporaries. Meg is determined to remain forever lithe and to continue to enjoy a large margin of aerobic power.

Meg recognizes the relationship between habitual physical activity and fitness. But daily energy output must be an effort of optimal level. A factory worker and a squash-playing bank clerk could have similar daily energy expenditures, yet entirely different aerobic ability. In *Nutrition, Physical Fitness, and Health,* the authors say, "There is little disagreement that variations in fitness (aerobic power) of 10 to 20 percent can be brought about in an individual, the magnitude depending on the initial level of fitness of the subject and the intensity of effort."[60]

Researchers find that there is no increase in working performance unless the heart rate exceeds 150 beats per minute. Thirty-minute efforts on a treadmill for four weeks will not do it if the pace is casual.[61] If you are above average in fitness, your exercise has to be correspondingly more vigorous to maintain that fitness. And that is why Meg walks fast. It is the energy expenditure complement she needs for her ballet exercises.

Nutrients and Performance

In an attempt to increase performance over the years, Meg learned about nutrients. The following information is part of her armamentarium:

- A number of ☆B vitamins☆ play a significant role in carbohydrate metabolism. According to the World Health Organization, a recommended daily intake of B vitamins is linked to energy expenditure, and the endurance athlete may require more of some vitamins than the average citizen.[62,63] There is also some loss of B vitamins in sweat.[64]
- ☆Vitamin C☆ deprivation leads to a reduction of work performance.[65] Russian researchers have attributed at least a part of the success of their athletes to the use of vitamin C supplements.[66] Other studies show that subjects receiving vitamin C supplements were able to perform better, the effect being similar to that of physical training,[67] and still others commented on a rapid recovery process following exercise in those given the vitamin.[68]
- The influence of ☆vitamin E☆ supplements upon performance is positive. One experimental group taking vitamin E suffered less loss of muscle strength than controls during three months of rigorous endurance training.[69] Another study shows a gain of maximum oxygen intake and a reduction of oxygen debt when vitamin E is administered to athletes exercising at high altitudes.[70]
- ☆Niacin☆ suppresses fatty acid and triglyceride levels when under □stress□.[71]

Meg has long since stopped proselytizing to the many practicing athletes who follow "special" and nutrient depleted dietary patterns. She knows that what they are doing is not in their best performance or health interest. They seem to focus upon relatively few dietary items. Aside from the fact that the diet is monotonous, a nonvaried diet runs the risk of concentrating specific contaminants and being deficient in specific nutrients. Valuable foods are often neglected, or even intentionally avoided because they are believed to be unsuitable for various physical exercises. Is this one of the reasons why former athletes have not done any better on the good-health continuum than the population at large? Athletes do not necessarily live longer or experience better cardiovascular health. There is no beneficial carry-over decades later. Meg is determined to be an exception.

As Meg checked her digital stopwatch to note the time and speed for distance covered, she exchanged smiles with "Dumpy." Dumpy looked so awkward as she slowly made her rounds, but she had a pleasant face.

AEROBNIC #5

Learning from the Media

Life for Sally Bender turned around because of an article in an anthropology magazine. This is what she tells people, but of course ideas favor the fertile mind. Sally was ready. Here's the article, written by Helen E. Fisher, anthropologist with the New York Academy of Sciences, and author of *The Sex Contract.*

During ☆**exercise**☆ blood bathes your skin and gums. Fluids wash your eyes. Nerves stimulate your muscles. Connective tissues massage your internal organs. Rhythmic breathing patterns relax your mind. With steady movement billions of your body cells are stimulated to take in clean substances and discard garbage. This refreshment the human body craves. [I know I have lots of body garbage to get rid of, but I thought it was ice cream my body craved.]

Why? Because steady daily exertion became essential to human life millions of years ago and through hundreds of centuries our bodily machinery has come to require exercise for health. [Don't I move around enough cleaning, cooking, shopping?] It all began over six million years ago when our first ancestors were forced from the fast disappearing trees of Africa to start a new life on the ground. Their food was scarce and their predators, the lions and leopards, roamed at will. So gradually they adopted an entirely new stand— bipedalism, or walking on two legs instead of four. With this posture, their mouths were freed to communicate, their arms released to carry sticks and stones to protect themselves. But most important, their lower limbs became designed to move distances with ease.

Now our human forebears could walk miles through the grasslands, collecting small game here, gathering birds' eggs, fruit, or vegetables over there, then moving on to new water holes, nutting groves, or game trails to collect the evening meal. [So don't I go from the Supermart to the Bargain Barn to the Fruit Emporium?] By jogging they could traverse greater distances to scout for potential prey. By running they could track and fell large beasts. [Doesn't chasing my kids when they were little count for anything? They were like wild animals.] So with time those that walked quickly, jogged easily, and ran efficiently survived and reproduced—passing, over thousands of generations, the human need for exercise to our masses of today.

This is your heritage; you are built to move. So you deserve to buy yourself a present—a pair of running shoes. [Do they have bags to match?] Put them on in the early morning, after you come home from work, or whenever you have fifteen minutes in your day. Then *walk* around the block as fast as you can walk. [The neighbors will think I am going through some kind of phase, or that my car broke down.] Tomorrow take another *walk*. By the third day of this routine, your body will remind you to take that walk. You will *want* to walk. In a few weeks you may want to trot just a few steps in the middle of your walk. In a few months your body will take you for a speedy trip. Let your body follow its natural, ancient pattern for survival.[72]

Sally clipped the article and took it to bed with her, reviewing it each night for a week. When she decided to make the commitment, she shared the information with Tom, reading aloud. He was less than enthusiastic, muttering something about, "It'll be another venture you won't see through. But go ahead—I know you will anyway. Buy the shoes." Sally suggested they both embark on the exercise program, that he needed it more than she did. But Tom's energies were already focused on Johnny Carson and a few snores.

It took one more piece of literature to motivate Sally from mental commitment to action. This was a statement made by the editor of *Nutrition Reviews*, Dr. Robert E. Olson:

A significant impediment to attaining good health in America is physical sloth, the tendency to sit instead of stand, to ride instead of walk, and to watch instead of participate in sports activities of all kinds. . . . It is folly to recommend decreasing caloric intakes to correct for decreasing physical activity in order to achieve a "desirable body weight." Below 1500 calories per day, on which a great number of middle-aged women maintain body weights with an enlarged fat component, it is doubtful some of the requirements for essential nutrients can be met. . . . To all Americans, get on your feet and get going—for health and happiness.[73]

Sally's Campaign

Sally's latest effort at dieting ended in failure, as usual. She pasted a picture of a beautiful girl inside her refrigerator. She lost a pound or two initially, but during the same time, Tom peered inside the fridge so often, he *gained* a few pounds.

Ignoring her husband's pessimism about "carrying through," Sally invested in running shoes, warm-up outfits, rebounder (a small, trampoline-like exerciser), jump rope, stopwatch, and sweat shirts. (It is no wonder her family bought her a T-shirt on which was inscribed, "When the going gets tough, the tough go shopping.") Sally surprised not only her husband, but even herself—she did indeed carry through. She would never admit to Tom that a few of her purchases were unnecessary. She settled in with an old pair of slacks and sweat shirt, used the rebounder only on nasty days, never picked up the jump rope or warm-up suits, and could have done without the watch (but timed herself daily to justify its acquisition).

Sally's "move-the-body" campaign had gotten off to a slow start. If walking was thwarted by rain, she would find it hard to get going again the next day. If she didn't walk on a Thursday, she would give herself the week-end off, vowing to continue on Monday. Monday came and went. It would take a week or two before she got going again. After two months of off-again-on-again-off-again, Sally drew up a contract. She actually wrote the following proclamation:

FOR THE NEXT NINETY DAYS I WILL WALK DAILY.
NO EXEMPTIONS. NO WEEK-END PASSES.
NO INCLEMENT WEATHER DISPENSATION.

By the end of the second contractual week, Sally was addicted. Nothing could prevent her from meeting the terms of her pledge. As she walked around the track, she projected to next year, at which time she envisioned a fifteen-pound weight loss, maybe more. She fantasized about being at cocktail parties, looking svelte, wearing any one of the dresses hanging in back of her closet, long since too small. Better yet—she dreamed of buying a new outfit in the *junior* department.

Sally began to feel better and better and better. As her health and well-being mounted, she tried to motivate Tom. Nothing she could say was convincing. She began to wonder if, in fact, Tom didn't want to get well. Did he enjoy the family's special pampering, elicited because of his high blood pressure, diabetes, and arthritis? Years back, at the onset of some of his symptoms, Sally accused him of being overconcerned. His children teased him. "Don't worry, Dad, if you die at an early age, we'll have your tombstone inscribed:

NOW WE BELIEVE HE WASN'T A HYPOCHONDRIAC

In spite of his complaints, Tom was able to laugh at himself along with his family. His favorite joke was: "I went to the doctor and told him I was sure I was dying from a serious liver disease. The doctor told me I would never know if I had liver disease because with that ailment there is no discomfort. So I said to the doctor, 'See, those are my exact symptoms.'"

Sally hoped her progress would inspire Tom. She wished his doctor would reinforce her proddings. Sally is not alone in her plea for recognition of the mutual importance of exercise, health, and medicine. An editorial in *Lancet*, Britain's prestigious medical journal, made an impassioned statement about concern at the contrast between the rapidly increasing public interest in exercise compared to the apathy, even antipathy, shown by many doctors.[74]

Sally was imaginative and, in anecdotal form, tried to impart the information she was gathering, hoping for Tom's attention:

- A man ran for a bus and had a heart attack. He should have been able to shunt more blood to his leg muscles. Instead, a large portion of his blood went to nonworking muscles in his arms or who knows where, but not his legs, because of poor circulation, because he didn't ☆exercise☆. So his heart had to pump twice as much blood as that of his healthy neighbor's, who was also running for the same bus.[75] The neighbor, who ☆**exercised**☆, was fine.

"Tom, are you listening?"
"I'm listening. I walk in the factory all day."
"It's not the same, and you know it."

- A woman thought she was exercising when she opened and closed her hand very rapidly. (Her doctor told her she had poor circulation in her hands.) She strengthened her hand muscles, but she didn't do much for over-all circulation. The larger the number of muscle groups exercised, the more oxygen the heart and circulation must deliver.[76]
- A lady had insomnia, and didn't want to take sedatives anymore. So she exercised. Vigorous exercise causes the release of hormones

called prostaglandins. These wonderful hormones promote sleep—without drugs. How do you like how clever your body is?[77]

"If you want me to go walking, I just developed a headache."

- Your doctor should do aerobics. He's too fat. So he plays tennis once in awhile. That's not aerobics. Aerobics is not *start* and *stop*. Aerobics is *steady*. If he walked for half an hour, he would begin to burn fat. And he should know that unused muscles degenerate rapidly and the inside of those muscles become larded with fat.[78]
- Two men did the same amount of moving around in a day. One had lower cholesterol and lower blood pressure. The difference is that one moved around in his factory, the other guy's activity was associated with leisure time.[79]

Tom responded with, "And I have news for you. Forced exercise will not decrease my blood pressure. That's been proved with rats.[80] But I am tired. And my doctor knows what's best."

"If your doctor knows what's best, why are you so tired all the time?"

"You want me to do something I hate, so I can live longer doing something I hate?"

Sally knew that Tom was right. If he went with her against his will, the stress would cause a lower level of oxygen uptake.[81] Some of his statements were valid, but Sally was convinced that Tom's attitude would change if he came out with her just once or twice. His resistance was frustrating.

Sally admired "The Couple." They looked compatible and happy. Even their children, who joined them on week-ends, appeared to be less pesky than most grade-school kids.

AEROBNICS #6 AND #7

Finding Time and Getting It Back

A news flash announced that a ball player signed a contract for $1 million. Jim Weiner playfully threw a football to his nine-year-old son and said, "If I see you touching that book again, I'll punish you." Of course Jimmy Junior knew his Dad was kidding. He also knew that exercise would bring more oxygen to his brain cells and boost his intellectual performance. His parents had told him so.

Despite the fact that most children are naturally active, Jane and Jim believe that their example of being involved in structured physical ☆activity☆ will help foster lifelong habits for their children. Michael Kamen, education consultant, says:

Children tend to do what we *do* rather than what we *say*, much to our frustration. When exercise is an important and enjoyable part of your life, it should enhance a child's interest and participation. Invite your children to join you in your physical activity. It can be a pleasant family time away from the old television set.

Forcing a child to exercise, especially when you are not modeling that behavior, won't promote the "fitness" attitude you would like your child to develop. Encourage, invite, and above all *show* your child that physical activity is important to you.[82]

Jane and Jim had to learn the hard way, and late in life: they did not move their bodies aerobically until age thirty, a couple of years ago. Their children would be different. Setting an example was their gift to the next generation.

Restoring the energy of their youth and the desire to lose a few pounds initiated interest in sports. A few trial and error programs of running, tennis, walking, rebounding, and rope jumping settled down to rebounding during inclement weather, occasional rope jumping, and walking most of the time.

The children love the rebounder and use it daily. Unfamiliar with rebounding until a friend described its advantages, they are now staunch advocates of this three-foot, circular, trampoline-like apparatus. Rebounding offers the benefits of jogging with less ▭**stress**▭ on muscles, ligaments, tendons, and organs of the body. Weight-bearing may be relieved as much as 85 percent as you rebound at your own pace on a walking, jogging, or running level. You can listen to music or even watch TV on the rebounder. You rebound in the privacy of your home, with no one witnessing your rolls of fat sloshing up and down.

But Jane and Jim also know the benefit of getting outdoors, of the value of natural light bathing skin, of that same light entering eyes and stimulating the pineal gland. Since their schedules are hectic and, like most people, time is at a premium, exercising outdoors attracted them.

Running proved disastrous. Jane's ankle went out, Jim's back went out, so running went out. Fast walking suited them both. Eventually, they reached their peak walking performance. They discovered that it was easier to intensify work by increasing incline rather than speeding up pace. They included hills and grades in their walk to the track.

One of their primary objectives had been weight reduction, and they learned that changes are largest when substantial amounts of energy are expended for some months. Perhaps for this reason long periods of vigorous walking do more to reduce body fat than brief sessions of jogging.[83] Although fat loss continues for more than a year when physical activity is increased,[84] a few months of vigorous training can correct most of the fat accumulation that occurs over the lifespan of an average person.[85]

Jane and Jim read that if you exercise just before your evening meal, you'll be more likely to lose a larger percentage of body fat than if you exercise at other times of the day. Ordinarily, metabolism slows down as the day wears on. But aerobics speeds things along.[86] What with the children's needs and dinner preparations, to say nothing of the fatigue experienced after a long day, the before-dinner routine did not work.

They tried lunch-hour exercise breaks and evening trials. Nothing succeeded as well as the discipline of getting up early in the morning, which is the one consistent time in most people's lives. It is not as easy to make up excuses and skip workouts if routinely planned for the A.M. Besides, Jane and Jim found it's a barter deal because they get their time back: on days that they exercise they require less sleep.

The Lactate Lament

At the outset of the exercise program, Jane's time around the track was shorter than Jim's. She had pains in her legs. Annoyed with the handicap, she learned about exercise discomfort: her ability to dispose of lactate (also known as lactic acid), generated by working muscles, was not as efficient as her husband's, and that's why she had pain. It has been theorized that lactic acid is a waste product from the chemical reaction which triggers working muscles and broken muscle tissue.[87] Another theory suggests that lactic acid is being burned for fuel.[88] It has also been stated that lactic acid has a chelating effect—that it binds with toxic minerals and calcium deposits, helping to remove them from the body. Since lactic acid exerts its beneficial effects as long as it is present in the circulating blood, the length of time of aerobic exercise, more than the intensity, is significant. (Another reason for longer walks rather than shorter runs.)[89] A tense muscle also gives off lactic acid.[90]

In any case, the rate of clearance of lactate is correlated with physical fitness, and either training or dietary changes augment both physical fitness and lactate clearance. With training, the body develops the capability of dealing with the process. As for the mechanisms of the nutritional manipulation, they are not clear, but high ☆**complex carbohydrate**☆ diets are recommended, with abstinence from simple sugars.

Jane's determination to keep up with Jim inspired her to improve her diet. In a short time, the pains stopped. Now and then she jumps rope on the rebounder. Rope jumping helps to trim legs, thighs, and hips, and to strengthen feet, ankles, and wrists. It improves balance, agility, and coordination. The rhythmic turning of the rope exercises her upper body. And, of course, as with the fast walking, there is a steady increase in the use of oxygen.

The children have responded favorably to the discipline of exercise. When they join Jane and Jim on week-end mornings, their parents' "walker's high" is more elevated than ever.

The children have noticed and questioned the sagacity of "Handsome Man Always Dripping Wet," who runs around the track as though he is being chased by a lion.

AEROBNIC #8

The Obligatory Runner

The "cowboy" is Keith Cummings. If Hollywood is searching for a type A personality who is a successful, top-level, □**stressed**□ executive, Keith fits the bill. He is a □**two-pack-daily**□, jet-set, □**three-martini**□ man, but is beginning to think about life-style changes.

Keith is on his way to becoming a fanatical runner. He started running when a girlfriend teased him about his paunch and about the dinner he had prepared for her. He had soaked a chicken all night in brandy, basted it with sherry, sprinkled it with vermouth, and put rum sauce in the dressing. "This chicken," she said, "is going to climb out of the oven and join Alcoholics Anonymous. Who needs it?" She added the final blow: "If you don't do something about your weight soon, you'll have more chins than a Chinese telephone directory." His extraordinarily high self-expectation and fear of projecting an image that was less than perfect motivated him to reduce liquor intake and start running. The running became an obsession. On days he cannot run he is depressed and anxious.

Keith is training for his first marathon. He runs at least fifty miles a week, ignoring and even denying several physical warnings. By assuming an identity as a runner, accented by his garb and gear, Keith is provided with a sense of self and a feeling of control he has never experienced before. Any dietary indiscretions are now redeemed by running longer and harder. He is consistently overlooking physiological needs. The alcohol and cigarette intake are being diminished—slowly—and he no longer strives to keep up with the "Dow Joneses." Now it's the fast runners. He is developing a heightened commitment to the sport, drawing his sword against body fat. He had always believed the best things in life are free, but now he no longer complains that the next best things are so expensive. Running is best, and next best. Running is everything, and cures everything. Fat is evil.

Keith thought he read somewhere that ▫**caffeine**▫ can improve athletic endurance by increasing the use of fat for energy. He upped his coffee intake, not entirely sure why.

Three doctors at the University of Arizona Health Sciences Center in Tucson have noted that "obligatory runners" like Keith resemble anorexic women in many ways. They have similar personality characteristics such as inhibition of anger, denial of potentially serious debility, tendency toward depression. The runners report subjective "highs." A point of interest is that anorexic patients are young women and the obligatory runners are often mature men. The doctors' explanation for this is:

The test of male physical effectiveness, which is closely related to vocational and sexual effectiveness, occurs in adulthood when careers stabilize and physical or sexual prowess begins to decline noticeably. The man with an uncertain identity and low self-esteem may experience exaggerated anxiety about physical ineffectiveness. The obligatory runner's solution to this problem would be to deny the decline in strength through a fanatic devotion to physical prowess. . . . Men of approximately age 40 become excessively or exclusively preoccupied with physical fitness after an often trivial threat to their physical well-being. . . . Anorexia and obligatory running are comparable to religious fanaticism or "workaholism" in that the pathology resides in the intensity and exclusiveness with which the adaptation is maintained.[91]

As Keith galloped around the track, he amused himself with the thought that the world could make better use of graffiti on lavatory walls. Time spent in bathrooms might represent untapped educational resources. His toilet posters would read:

RUNNERS HAVE MORE FUN
RUN FOR YOUR LIFE
GET A RUN FOR YOUR MONEY
RUNNERS LOVE HEAVY BREATHING
HAVE A RUN OF LUCK
RUN CIRCLES AROUND YOUR FRIENDS
DON'T RUN AMUCK: JUST RUN
DON'T BE PUT OUT OF THE RUNNING

The thing that hath been, it is that which shall be; and that which is done, is that which shall be done: and there is no new thing under the sun.

- The Bible
  Arise, and take up thy bed and walk.
- 1400s—Desiderius Erasmus
  "Before supper walk a little:
  After supper do the same."
- 1800s—Charles Dickens
  "Walk and be healthy. The best way to lengthen out our days is to walk steadily and with a purpose."
- May, 1983—International Exercise Panel, England
  "Man was built for exercise. There would be huge benefits to public health if the general level of participation in exercise could be increased."[92]
- July, 1983—Morris County, New Jersey
  Women at work in an office decided to spend their fifteen-minute breaks doing simple ☆**exercises**☆ to fight "sedentary spread" and to boost morale. But the women were told to cease the workouts and go back to drinking ▫**coffee**▫ during their breaks. The problem? Exercise is no coffee substitute because the county could be liable if anyone was injured while working out.[93]

CHAPTER 2

Image Projection

The centenarian was being honored on national television. The host asked, "If you had it to do over, what would you have done differently?" The 100-year-old answered, "If I had known I was going to live so long, I would have taken better care of myself."

BOB'S EYE VIEW OF FRIENDS AND NEIGHBORS

The Medicine Cabinet

"Our subways aren't safe, our streets aren't safe, our parks aren't safe, but under our arms and in our mouths we have complete protection." Bob was listening to the DJ on the radio as he slid the small mirrored door of his medicine cabinet to one side, exposing its contents. The comedian continued:

"I should have listened to my mother and gone to beauticians' school. Instead I had to become a nuclear physicist. I'm so unattractive that under the word 'ugly' in the dictionary they have my picture."

Bob suddenly wondered who was responsible for the misnomer, "medicine" chest. Sure, these units usually contain a bottle of aspirin, relief agents for stomach upset, outdated prescriptions, last season's suntan lotion, and possibly an antiseptic cream. But the get-well items are outnumbered by youth elixirs—products intended to cover up, minimize, reverse, or prevent any signs of aging or fading good looks. Wouldn't "Camouflage Cupboard" be a more accurate name?

> Beauty is not immortal. In a day,
> Blossom and June and rapture pass away."[1]

As Bob turned the couplet over in his mind, he thought of the cosmetic industry and its advantage: beauty's impermanence.

Bob scanned the receptacles of his private collection, and saw:

> Hair tonic
> Hair spray
> Lip bleach (his wife's)
> Nail polish (his wife's)
> Underarm deodorant (his)
> Underarm deodorant (hers)
> Perfumes
> Hand cream
> Myriad makeup mixtures
> After-shave lotion
> Band-aids
> Nail file
> Combs

The ultimate of all nonaging potions—*feeling terrific*—could not be captured in any container, thought Bob, as his mind wandered to a patient he had seen yesterday. The patient had an advanced state of cancer and looked ten years older in only two weeks. This, of course, is an extreme case of accelerated aging.

It is true that many diseases do not necessarily produce illness, and some features of illness—that is, the manifestations or symptoms of distress—may be independent of disease.[2] Bob's clinical observations, however, have taught him that when symptoms are present, whether caused by serious illness or temporary lack of ☆**homeostasis**☆, the body reflects an overall "older" look. (Homeostasis is internal normalcy.) As stress is reduced, or disease eliminated, youthfulness returns. If we could only bottle health, or homeostasis, perhaps we could discard most of the contents of the camouflage cabinet.

Bob keeps a small medicine kit on hand in a cabinet underneath the sink. Some of the items were formerly kept in the medicine chest, but Bob discourages their use in his household. Should an emergency arise, the products are there. From time to time, he replenishes supplies. Among these are:

Cortisone ointment
Strong headache drugs
Pain killers
Ear clearers (for wax build-up)
Skin abrasion creams
Diarrhea remedies
Antiseptics for wounds
Anticough preparations
Antacids
Antibiotics
Mucous-drying compounds
Burn ointment ("Shouldn't we keep this in the kitchen?")
Baby powder containing hexachlorophene
Anticonvulsant

Bob is fully aware that the side effects of some of these □**drugs**□ are worse than any symptom they attempt to relieve. He can't fully explain why he keeps all of them on hand. (Medical school, drug-oriented training, perhaps.) Even baby powder, which appears innocent enough, may be lethal. A recent epidemic of skin poisoning in France affected a couple of hundred children, thirty-six of whom died. The source of the toxic agent was talcum powder which, because of a manufacturing error, contained high levels of hexachlorophene.[3] (Hexachlorophene has been banned in the U.S. But old containers abound in many American bathrooms.)

The urine of nurses working in oncology (cancer) wards can be more mutagenic (capable of changing the genetic code) than that of nurses in other units.[4] Absorption of chemotherapy drugs (which nurses have to mix and administer to patients) takes place in these health-care personnel either through the skin or through inhalation.[5]

Phenytoin, an anticonvulsant found in Dilantin, can lower folate levels in many patients taking this □**drug**□, which could have devastating effects, and promote anemia.[6] (Folate is a compound of the ☆**B vitamin**☆ complex.) But taking large amounts of folic acid to correct the deficiency may *induce* seizures. Elimination of seizures is the very reason the drug is administered in the first place.[7]

There are many other □**drug**□/☆**nutrient**☆ interactions. Even common aspirin can cause nutritional problems. Chronic use of salicylates (used in the manufacture of aspirin) has been shown both to decrease uptake of ☆vitamin C☆ in leukocytes (the body's defense cells) and impair the protein-binding ability of folate.[8]

In the *New England Journal of Medicine*, Hoffman La-Roche, Inc. brings nutrient/drug interactions home to doctors with full page ads defining some of the specific impacts. Among the interactions listed:

□Drug□	☆Vitamin☆ affected	Possible manifestation and mechanisms
Mineral Oil	A, D, K	Rickets
Cholestyramine [to lower cholesterol, such as Questran]	Folacin, B_{12}, A, D, K	Osteomalacia (Bone and muscular weakness)
Colchicine [for gouty arthritis]	B_{12}	Absorptive enzyme damage Damage to intestinal wall
Glutethimide [Doriden, for temporary insomnia]	D	Osteomalacia
Hydralazine [Apresoline, for hypertension]	B_6	Peripheral Nutropathy Increased excretion of vitamin/drug complex
Neomycin [Mycifradin, for diarrhea]	B_{12}, A	Damage to intestinal wall Binding of bile salts Intrinsic factor inhibition (necessary for B_{12} absorption)
Penicillamine [Cuprimine, for rheumatoid arthritis]	B_{12}	Peripheral neuropathy (Nervous disorders of extremities)

▫**Drug**▫	☆**Vitamin**☆ affected	Possible manifestation and mechanisms
Potassium Chloride [Kayciel, to compensate for drug-induced deficiency]	B_{12}	Decreased ileal pH (Condition of body fluids)
Salicylates [aspirin]	Folacin, C, K	Decreased protein binding Decreased uptake in thrombocytes (blood platelets) and leukocytes (white blood cells)
Sulphasalazine [Azulfidine, for ulcerative colitis]	Folacin	Decreased absorption
Tetracycline	C	Increased excretion

As professional as his home cache of pharmacopia may be, Bob knows his supply would be found wanting if compared with that of some of his nonmedical neighbors. The thought of anyone having quantities of medicines so easily available, even if the substances are sold "over the counter," disturbs him. Not that he feels that the drug user necessarily requires doctor's supervision. His attitude stems mainly from his belief that most common ailments disappear if you let nature take its course, and from the fact that *there are no* ▫**drugs**▫ *without side effects. Only ineffective drugs can be safe.*[9]

On the Spot Diagnosing

Bob shaved and dressed and made his appearance at a neighborhood gathering. His dying cancer patient was on his mind. He found himself working overtime, still reaching out with a profusion of antennae, noticing such things as cracks in the corners of someone's mouth, hair that had lost its luster, complexions that were pale. Subtle skin differences and even posture changes were obvious to him. As he assessed friends and neighbors, he silently assigned nutrition deficiencies. His diagnoses were as swift as his observations.

Mary. Her hair had no natural shine, and an attempt at "teasing"—an effort to conceal the fact that it was dull, dry, and sparse—was no distraction for Bob. He guessed that it would also "pluck" far too easily, and concluded that Mary might be in trouble, with multiple, coexistent nutrient deficiencies, including protein-calorie depletion—probably the result of extreme food limitation to keep her weight down. Mary is a secret noneater. She thought about food so much that when a friend confided that she was having an affair, she asked, "Who's catering?" (Oliver Wendell Holmes said, "Beauty is the index of a larger fact than wisdom.")

Ann. If the eyes have it, Ann's didn't. What they did have was pale conjunctivitis—redness and fissuring of the eyelid corners. This signaled possible iron, niacin, riboflavin, and pyridoxine deficiency. Ann would benefit by including ☆**liver**☆ in her diet, or taking desiccated liver tablets, which supply both iron and ☆**B complex**☆. ☆**Ascorbic acid**☆ enhances iron absorption. Ann was expendiing a lot of energy (and probably nutrients) while engaged in a heated discussion. Politics or religion? As Bob closed in on the group, he realized the issue was even more pressing: "Where does one get a plumber on the week-end?"

Joe. Redness and swelling of his lips denoted niacin and riboflavin deficiencies. (Again, these are components of ☆**B complex**☆.) Joe announced that he was celebrating his fortieth birthday, and he had every intention of living up to the cliché that life begins at forty. A wise guy retorted, "So do double chins and wrinkles."

Arnie. Arnie's "gummy" smile facilitated the assessment that he might have a serious ☆**ascorbic acid**☆ deficiency: His gums were spongy looking. He had just returned from an extensive business trip and boasted that all in one day he enjoyed breakfast in London, lunch in New York, dinner in San Francisco. "But my baggage was in Tokyo." He laughed heartily at his own joke, exposing his nutritional faults.

Julie. Bob overheard Julie discussing her new "put-on" nails. "It's so easy," said Julie. "The fake nails hide my short, rotten nails, which are so brittle and full of ridges. They break all the time." Iron deficiency, concluded Bob silently. If she had complained of white spots on her nails, the diagnosis might be zinc bankruptcy. As Bob passed this group, he was stopped. "Bob, is there a medical term for brittle nails?" "Sure," the good doctor said, smiling. "It's called 'having brittle nails.' "

John. His skin looked dry and flaky. ☆**Vitamin A**☆ deficiency; insufficient unsaturated and essential fatty acids, all too common in America today. Skin is nourished by capillaries which are so minute that blood cells go through them in single file. Nutritional deficiencies close these pathways, creating dull, dry, listless and finely wrinkled surfaces. Skin is at the end of the line, reflecting the condition of internal organs. Bob mused that he might miss these symptoms in women: the worse the condition of their skin, the greater the application of makeup. A solution that could save everyone a lot of grief would be to cover all mirrors with vaseline.

Connie. Dark circles under her eyes. This could be inadequate caloric intake, or allergy. Connie did not need the cigarette in her mouth to reveal that she was a ▫**smoker**▫. Bob could always tell, cigarette in evidence or not. Even the skin-care product guaranteed to take wrinkles out of prunes would not help Connie.

Bob had attended a medical meeting recently. The audience began to nod, half asleep, as the speaker droned on about the dangers of smoking. Lung cancer. Heart disease. Suddenly everyone came alive. It causes wrinkles! This disturbing effect appears in both men and women after age 30. But the real clincher is that smokers in the 40-to-49-year group are likely to be as prominently wrinkled as nonsmokers who are twenty years older. ("You've come a long way, pruneface.")[10]

Mollie. At first glance Bob thought Mollie was pregnant. After spending a few minutes with her, he realized that she was edematous (having an accumulation of fluid in the tissues, characterized by puffiness or swelling). Bob's traditional lessons taught him that this may be caused by obstruction of veins or lymphatic vessels, or the condition could be generalized as kidney disease. His newly acquired nutritional insights suggest edema may be the result of food sensitivity.[11] The term "edema" is often used for "overhydration," but these are different conditions.[12] Mollie would be a challenging patient.

The message of the keynote speaker at his medical school graduation stayed with him: "Half of what you have learned will prove to be invalid. The trouble is, you don't know yet which half." Mollie was telling a joke. "My doctor told me that sex prevents arthritis. When I shared this information with my husband, he said, 'You don't have arthritis.' So I said 'Don't you believe in preventive medicine?' "

Lorraine. She has an exquisite tan. But then Lorraine *always* has a beautiful tan. As Lorraine explains, "If we lived in the days of □sun worship□, I'd be the most religious person in the world." Bob saw the first telltale signs of overexposure: Her freckles were growing larger. He hoped she knew about PABA (para-aminobenzoic acid), which is a component of folic acid, but is often classed as a separate vitamin. PABA absorbs ultraviolet energy, thereby blocking its damaging effects to the skin. Dietary supplementation of PABA may lessen the susceptibility to sunburn in those persons easily affected. Vitamin B_6 taken orally is sometimes even more effective. It facilitates tanning.

Taking fewer baths is advice Bob won't even discuss, because he knows it will go unheeded. Bathing dries the natural oils of the skin. In addition, vitamin D, manufactured in the body as a result of daylight exposure, is absorbed gradually. You run the risk of absorbing soap, rather than vitamin D, when you bathe too soon after being out in the sun.[13,14,15]

All these trumpet calls could have been brought about by unfavorable environmental conditions and/or inadequate nutritional status. Sometimes they are flags of more serious diseases. Bob recognizes that no single indicator is significant in itself, and also that nutrients work synergistically—one vitamin, mineral, hormone, and enzyme depending on other vitamins, minerals, hormones, and enzymes. He often refers to the inimitable Roger Williams (renowned for having called to the world's attention the fact that we are all uniquely different biologically). Roger Williams says:

The need for phenylalanine is decreased if tyrosine is supplied; the need for methionine is decreased if cystine is supplied; and the need for tryptophane hinges in part on how much niacinamide is in the diet.[16]

The irony for Bob is that every person in attendance at this gathering has spent at least some time in front of the bathroom mirror, applying this or that balm, salve, ointment, cosmetic, liniment, poultice, oil, garnish, polish, or powder—pulled from their sundry camouflage cabinets—intent, not only on looking his or her best, but on

looking as young as possible. Correcting nutritional deficiencies, however, happens to be the master stroke. And it doesn't come in a bottle.

Bob's Paper Chase

Bob is hard-pressed to research the nutrition science—the kind he
can back up with credibility. Although medical journals are beginning
to fill with studies and reports of nutrient/health correlations, final
interpretations involve sifting through differences and controversies.
This requires the judgment of Solomon.

One disadvantage is the eighty-year average latency period (with
a thirty-five year standard deviation) from the time a study is reported
in the literature to the time it becomes common, everyday knowledge.
This built-in lag exceeds the age of contemporary nutrition itself.
Contemporary nutrition looks at degenerative disease as that which may
be internal, but is impacted by environment (including diet). This
philosophy is a babe in arms, born only twenty years ago. Shift takes
time—sometimes thirty-five to fifty or more years of time.[17]

Another bottleneck arises from difficulties in filtering through studies
in an effort to pull out those which may be misleading. For example,
Dr. Jeffrey Bland, professor of biochemistry at the University of Puget
Sound, cites the details of an article which "proved" that megadoses
of vitamin C (1000 milligrams daily) had no effect in lowering cholesterol. More careful scrutiny of the report reveals, however, that men
chosen for this study had cholesterol levels of 174 at the outset of the
research. A cholesterol level of 174 is uniquely low. (The average
cholesterol value in this country is 225.) Previous research has shown
that vitamin C lowers cholesterol if the level is high to begin with. In
fact, states Dr. Bland, if the cholesterol level is 350, it may be lowered
as much as 70 points. If it is 250, there could be a 20-point drop. But
there is no decline if the level is already low. (This is another example
of how nature tends to the normal.) It appears that the protocol—the
game plan of a scientific study—which was used to "disprove" the cholesterol lowering/ascorbic acid theory, was preselected to determine the
outcome of the study. The subjects were obviously not chosen at ran-
dom.[18,19] It is this kind of sophistry that infuriates Bob.

Given these difficulties, Bob is an anecdote collector. One story
does not validate a theory, but he finds personal experiences of other
doctors (and his own) to be of great benefit. He believes doctors learn

more from their impressions and observations of patients than they do from controlled doubleblind studies, which, in addition to shortcomings already stated, often ignore the fact that we function as biological human beings.

The classic example of how doctors really learn is inherent in the story of green yogurt. A doctor teaches his patients how to make their own yogurt. A few days later one patient calls and says, "Doctor, my yogurt turned green." The doctor says, "Oh, how surprising. You must have done something wrong." A few days later another patient calls and says, "Doctor, my yogurt turned green." The doctor says, "Well, that happens on occasion." Finally, a third patient calls with the same complaint. "Oh," says the doctor, "that's a common occurrence."

Bob has mentally filed anecdotes told by his colleagues and reported in medical literature:

Psoriasis presents a dilemma. There is no ideal treatment. A therapy called PUVA, which entails the use of psoralen, a drug that is activated by light, combined with exposure to ultraviolet light, has been used with reports of good results. But adverse effects are being noted. Patients on the treatment may suffer visual field defects. They may experience tunnel vision and photophobia.[20] (Tunnel vision is a reduction in visual field, similar to looking through a long tunnel or tube. Photophobia is abnormal visual sensitivity to light.)

Better news comes from one doctor who reports excellent results after five years of treatment, which includes the elimination of acid foods. This means no fruit (especially citrus), coffee, tomatoes, soda, or pineapple. In addition, no nuts, corn, or milk are allowed. There are no side effects and the therapy is simple, easily administered, and reasonably effective. The theory is that your own gut bacteria, which must absorb what you put in your intestines, excrete drug-type eruptions because gut microorganisms manufacture □**drug**□-like or toxic substances when you ingest certain items.

The doctor added that he found this regimen helpful in patients with various other skin problems.[21]

Skin Rashes are proliferating. Searching for contributing factors requires the skill of Sherlock Holmes, the medical expertise of Quincy, and the genius of Einstein. One possibility may be skin reactions to □**alcohol**□-containing topical products, especially when patients are taking particular □**drugs**□, which interact with □**alcohol**□. Absorption of many chemicals is enhanced by heat, friction, and moisture, so that showering with a beer-containing shampoo, or rubbing on colognes, after-shave lotions, and sunscreen lotions may produce reactions.[22] This also demonstrates the synergistic effects of chemicals—the substances in the topical applications with the substances in a ☐drug☐. Bob has learned to question carefully when any patient shows him a rash. The first question is, "What ☐drugs☐ are you taking?"

Melanoma, a skin tumor containing the dark pigment melanin, is often easily remedied. If the melanoma metastasizes (spreads rapidly), it is more serious. This kind of tumor may start in a black mole. Bob is never content to remove the offending tumor. He wants to get at causes, the only way he knows to prevent recurrence.

There is an association between exposure to ☐**fluorescent**☐ lighting, office work, and an excess of malignant melanoma. Polychlorinated biphenyls (PCBs) have been associated with melanoma and other cancers. PCBs are mainly used in closed electric components, such as the small capacitors found in fluorescent light installations, air conditioners, and data processing screen terminals. An investigation in Norway showed increased PCB concentrations in the office atmosphere. Especially high PCB levels were detected in kitchens, offices, and laboratories. On a day with burnout of a fluorescent light ballast, the PCB levels were found to be over fifty times higher than normal for that room, and levels remained high for three to four months.[23]

The link between malignant melanoma and exposure to fluorescent lighting has been confirmed by the National Institute for Occupational Safety and Health (NIOSH) at the Department of Environmental Medicine, New York University Medical Center.[24]

Bob encourages patients to change their fluorescent bulbs wherever possible. Full-spectrum fluorescent bulbs are available; incandescent bulbs do not present the same problems.

French Vanilla Frostbite was the focal point of an interesting story. A colleague of Bob's told him about a young patient who had cold sores which were truly sores from the cold. The cold sores on the lips of an eighteen-month-old had come from an enthusiastic relationship with a French vanilla ice-cream cone. The child did not remove her mouth from the treat for an hour and a half. Over the next two days, the affected areas progressed in a manner typical of local frostbite, with blistering occurring on both upper and lower lips. Although

Bob has not yet had occasion to diagnose French vanilla frostbite, he did see a child with popsicle pollution. Since the lesions broke out several days after this child had come in contact with the cold object, the parents were impressed with Dr. Smith's diagnosis when he traced the malady back to the popsicles.[25]

Petechia, a pinpoint, nonraised, perfectly round, purplish red spot caused by small hemorrhages within the skin, may form about the ankles of joggers, especially if they have been previously unexercised. Basketball players, with sudden starts and stops, are known to get petechia on the soles of their feet.[26]

Sunglass Syndrome was described by one doctor, and sure enough, Bob had a patient with similar symptoms. Annoying sensations beneath the eyes and over the cheeks, which gradually progressed to involve the nose (where the sensation was one of numbness), were caused by wearing large sunglasses for several hours every day. The numbness was also experienced while brushing and water-picking the teeth. It is suggested that large sunglasses exert pressure on nerve endings, causing the discomfort.[27]

Cardiopulmonary Resuscitation (CPR) is a technique Bob encourages patients to learn. But he cautions the resuscitator to clear respiratory passages of any foreign bodies that may be transmitted to the poor victim. The case of the missing dental bridge is rather humorous, and Bob does not anticipate its recurrence. It's another story he has filed away, just in case. A 60-year-old man collapsed at a social function, and received CPR from the bartender. After the patient was hospitalized, serious complications developed, which were eventually traced to a foreign object: the dental bridge belonging to the bartender, which was lost during the mouth-to-mouth resuscitation.[28]

Bob thought jokes about objects being left in a patient during an operation were ridiculous, until he learned that "many a truth is in fact said in jest." One of his favorite silly jokes is about a man who discovered that a sponge was left in his tummy after an operation. When asked if he was in pain, the man said, "No, but am I thirsty!"

Bob collects his stories and his patients benefit. His greatest challenge is changing basic behavior. To accomplish this goal, he has found it necessary to offer a recognizable reward. This might, for example, be in terms of appearance, rather than health. Very few people decide

"It is healthier for me to replace the bulbs and lighting style in my house or office, and it is better to prepare a ☆**bean**☆ dish tonight instead of lamb chops, so I will do it." However, the prospect of a more beautiful complexion may be the incentive. When correlations are made between the image one projects and the need for change, then and only then does Bob have his patient's attention (not necessarily cooperation). But at least it's a start. His ultimate objective is to make healthful eating easy, without perpetual anxiety about good nutrition.

BEN AND KITCHEN CUPBOARD CURES

Feeling Young at Any Age

Have you not a moist eye? a dry hand? a yellow cheek? a white beard? a decreasing leg? an increasing belly? is not your voice broken? your wind short? your chin double? your wit single? and every part about you blasted with antiquity? and will you yet call yourself young? Fie, fie![29]

Yes, William, I call myself young because I *feel* young.

Ben studied his face in the mirror. When he first memorized these lines in his Shakespeare reciting days, the thought of Ben Carpenter acquiring the classic stance, gait, and countenance of an older person was a thousand years away. But looking back, those Shakespeare days were only yesterday.

He accepts his mortality, but asks: Couldn't there be a more harmonious decline of organ reserve, rather than such a glaring presentation of aging? Must chins jut forward, elbows stick out, backs be slightly bent? "In all these decades, the only thing that hasn't gone up in value," Ben declares, "is me!" And to his grandchildren he comments, "I'm so old I remember when toilet paper came in only one color." Or, "When a fellow worker said he was going to retire, it meant he was going to bed."

But inside, Ben does not *feel* old. He firmly believes that you do not stop laughing because you grow old, but that you grow old because you stop laughing. Ben's succinct words are, "He who laughs, lasts." Ben knows he looks younger than his years. His latest humorous story is about a recent medical examination. The doctor said to him, "You'll surely live to be eighty." "But I am already eighty!" The doctor said, "See, what did I tell you?"

Ben opened his medicine cabinet. He never touched or looked at the items on the left-hand side:

> Cough mixture
> Nasal spray
> Joint pain rub
> Oxide ointment for burns
> Witch hazel

If he kept these things on hand, he reasoned, he would never have to use them. Superstition, maybe, but it worked. He stored his toothpaste and shaving equipment on the right-hand side. Ben was old enough to regard any pleasant smelling lotion as feminine. In his growing-up days, only women used perfumed substances. He resisted medication, even when prescribed. His nostrums were in his kitchen:

Honey. Ben never eats honey—it's too sweet for his taste. He stores it to accelerate wound healing, a trick handed down in his family for generations. He simply applied the honey to any cut or open wound. This folk remedy provoked amusement and teasing on the part of his children, until his granddaughter, a medical student, offered scientific validation. She learned from the *American Journal of Surgery* that unboiled honey, applied topically, speeds the healing process due to its energy-producing properties, its hygroscopic (moisture attracting or absorbing) effect on the wound, and its bactericidal (bacteria destroying) activity.[30]

Several researchers have suggested that ▫sugar▫ could be used as a nonspecific "universal" antimicrobial agent.[31] Doctors have pointed out, however, that the low pH (acidity) of commercial honey creates an instant unfavorable environment for bacterial growth which cannot be achieved by granulated sugar. The tissue dehydration caused by honey is rapid, and requires only twice-a-day application, as opposed to the need for more frequent additions of sugar to maintain a therapeutic level of water activity in the wound. If tissues become too dry with the use of honey, saline packs may be used.[32]

Aloe Vera Plant. The rest of America is catching up to Ben. Aloe vera plants adorn more gardens and kitchen windowsills than ever before. The aloe is best known for its healing properties. Although a folk remedy, it is used extensively in many commercial preparations. Whenever Ben needs to soothe a burn, reduce pain of any skin injury, lessen an inflammation (including a persistent one that flares up between two of his toes), or prevent sunburn peeling, he breaks off a piece of this spineless, fleshy cactus, and splits the portion of the spiky leaf he has severed. He either scrapes out the mucilaginous pulp and applies it to the ravaged area, or uses the leaf itself as the bandage. In addition to relieving pain, facilitating healing, and serving as an antibiotic, aloe appears to encourage regeneration of normal skin cells, minimizing unsightly scars.

History reveals that Cleopatra used aloe gel as a face mask, replenishing lost moisture and helping to attain a soft and radiant complexion. Japanese used it to treat survivors of the Hiroshima and Nagasaki bombings. Columbus mentioned its medicinal uses in his ship's log. Hunters in Africa coat themselves with aloe to reduce human perspiration and odor, enabling them to approach game without detection.[33] Two thousand years ago it was reported as a treatment for blisters, itching, and even hemorrhoids.

When Ben purchases his "living medicine chest" and "cosmetic kit," he looks for a mature plant, at least three years old. It takes that many years for the aloe plant to develop its active ingredients, which, by the way, are nonallergenic and noncarcinogenic. If the plant is purchased at a commercial garden nursery, it should be rinsed thoroughly. Nurseries use sprays indiscriminately.

Ben claims that his aloe vera plant is his way of beating the establishment. The major theme of medieval alchemy was the quest for transforming materials into gold. In the 1980s, this has been accomplished. In 1982, gold was reported at about $11.75 per gram.[34] An antibiotic developed in 1981 costs pharmacists $12.20 per gram. An antiinflammatory agent checks in at $55.50 per gram, while a popular hypertension drug sells for $120.00 per gram. Nitroglycerin at 5 cents a tablet ($5 per 100 tablets) costs $125 per gram, or $3,750 per ounce. Priced as it is delivered by unit dose in at least one local hospital, it costs $3,275 per gram, or $98,250 per ounce. (Perhaps investors should stockpile drugs instead of gold coins.) The question is, are these drugs worth more than their weight in gold?[35,36] Ben doesn't think so. Not when his aloe vera plant costs $3.50!

Ben explains that there have been times in ancient history when medicine was thought to be worth more than gold. As an example, when the tomb of Tutankhamen was opened, it was learned that thieves, some thousands of years before, had tunneled into the sacred dwelling, evading or bribing the ubiquitous royal tomb guardians and bypassing incredible Pharaonic treasures only to steal jars of unguents or medi-caments.[37] Inflation notwithstanding, the gold/drug relationship goes back to antiquity.

Oatmeal. Whenever Ben returns from family barbecues, filled with warm feelings and insect bites, he cooks oatmeal, places the cereal in a loose cheesecloth bag, and adds it to his bath water. His late wife, Ida, used to add honey to coarsely ground oatmeal. She scrubbed her face, or softened and protected her hands with the mixture. Oatmeal as a substitute for soap is still in everyday use in many parts of the world.[38]

Lemons. To soften foot calluses, Ben rubs lemon on his feet. If Ida had to sit awhile (which she rarely did, but maybe she was waiting for a cake to bake), she would dunk her elbows into the squeezed halves of lemon skins to bleach out rough and red spots. She rubbed the juice on her hands as a skin beautifier.[39] A taxi driver once told Ben that you can tell a woman's age by looking at her elbows. Not so with Ida!

Cayenne Pepper. This condiment, so forceful in foods, is very subtle within the body. It is a digestive aid, calling to arms all secret-ing organs. Ben adds a tiny pinch to many cooked or raw foods, even a dash to soup or tea.

If he senses an impending sore throat, he gargles with a mix of cayenne, salt, apple cider vinegar, and water. Cayenne becomes his liniment when added to alcohol and diluted with water. If he cuts himself while shaving, it is his styptic: a few grains stop bleeding al-most immediately. But his ace maneuver is its use for cold feet (liter-ally, cold feet). He sprinkles a combo of cayenne pepper and dusting powder into his shoes on blustery days. This is second only to placing your tootsies on your mate's warm back.[40]

Ice cubes. More than 2000 years ago, Hippocrates described the use of ice and snow packs as a presurgical local analgesic technique.[41] Ben applies ice to any area screaming out with sharp pain.

Ben's Friends; Ben's Memories

Ben has long since given up his efforts to get his contemporaries (the few who are left) to stop seeing all those doctors. One of his friends goes to a physician who arranges so many appointments for him with specialists, he sounds like a booking agent.

"Sure, I know, it was needed surgery; the doctor needed the money."

As Ben turned from the bathroom mirror, he could remember hearing Ida, as she looked into this same mirror, smiling and saying, "Beauty is but a flower, which wrinkles will devour."[42] And now Ben is saying: "Old as I am, for ladies' love unfit, the power of beauty I remember yet."[43]

MAN WITH BLUE CAP: NOW WE KNOW WHY

Only A Few Perfect Heads

Mike's medicine cabinet contains:

Head Start (protein for hair)
Vitamins for Hair (instructions: one tablet a day)
Solar Vita Hair: For Beautiful Hair (vitamins for hair, one tablet a day)
The Australian Three-Minute Miracle (a phytogenic/botanical deep penetrating hair reconstructor)
Thicket Special Formula (makes thin fine hair thicker)
H-Pantothen (containing pantothenic acid, biotin, and other nutrients reported to aid hair growth)
Valisone (no claims made, but ointment noted to stimulate hair growth[44])
Banfi Herbaria (a Hungarian product, not available in this country; obtained from a traveling friend; hair thickener)

Many of these products are of a vintage that would boost their price if they were wines. Mike hasn't discarded the hair-growth hope chest because the products have been resting on these shelves so long he doesn't "see" them anymore. Everything else in the cabinet concerns his teeth. His brother is a dentist, and has supplied him with:

Proxa-handle for stimulating the gingivae between teeth
Proxa-brush refills
A between-the-teeth brush
Kenalog in orabase (cortisone to cover oral sores)
Neosporin (ointment for skin lesions and sores)

Dental floss
Scalers to remove tartar from teeth

The funny little story that "God created only a few perfect heads, and the rest he covered with hair," has not been much solace to Mike. It would have been his preference to be among the less perfect. He does, however, find joy in the fact that male pattern baldness has been linked to increased excretion of male hormone.[45] And of course he enjoys quoting Shakespeare: "What he hath scanted men in hair, he hath given them in wit."[46]

Is It In the Genes?

Mike has finally given up examining his scalp for signs of hair growth each time he uses a product laced with innumerable promises. About 80 percent of the time, the no-hair genes are a present from Mom's side of the family. Mike questions the inherited theory in his case because his maternal grandfather was not bald, nor were either of his mother's grandfathers.

Mike has learned the following:

- The condition of hair reflects the condition of the body. Hair should be well nourished through capillaries and blood vessels fed by the bloodstream. If the blood is undernourished, then the hair becomes undernourished too.[47]
- Overactive sebaceous glands are considered a contributing cause of common baldness.[48] (Sebaceous glands are the oil-secreting skin glands.)
- Women are not exempt from the increasing affliction of baldness today. Thinning or early baldness is suffered by 15 to 20 percent of all females past adolescence. It is estimated that about 80 percent of the male population will eventually suffer hair loss. ☆**Nutritional**☆ deficiencies and ▢**pollution**▢ are additional culprits.[49]
- Oval-shaped heads have poorer circulation than other shapes, and consequently may have poorer hair growth.[50]
- ☆**Zinc**☆ is essential for hair growth, and copper is a zinc antagonist.[51]
- Biotin is a ubiquitous member of the vitamin ☆**B complex**☆. Deficiency has been produced by feeding large quantities of uncooked ☆**egg**☆ white. Biotin is found in egg yolks, but rendered unavailable because of avidin, found in raw egg whites. In test animals,

alopecia (baldness) and graying of fur occur when there is biotin deficiency. Although biotin deficiency is rare in humans, cases have been noted, and guess what: these people are bald. Administration of biotin promotes normal hair growth for people who do have biotin deficiency. It is suggested that this information will be an important clue to understanding and ultimately curing people with alopecia.[52,53]

One might conclude that eggs are excellent, but not necessarily in their raw state if used in quantity. And once again, nutrient interactions must not be overlooked: other nutrient deficiencies or excesses may play a significant role in improper biotin metabolism.

- Rare patients suffering from rickets also have alopecia. It is the hope of researchers that this knowledge will enhance understanding.[54] One wonders if the increase in alopecia and the decrease in use of cod-liver oil are related.

- Androgens (any substances possessing masculinizing activities, such as the testicular hormone) are known to cause scalp hair loss in men and women.[55] A 38-year-old man who had male pattern baldness since he was twenty was on a potent drug for hypertension. He had extensive scalp hair growth during this treatment, even while receiving additional androgen in another drug.[56] Despite the additional androgen, hair growth was stimulated. This is not a recommendation for the use of hypertension drugs, but just another bit of information to file away, emphasizing the complexity of biological processes.

As Mike remembers it, his first sign of trouble occurred when he put his head back on a pillow at age 21, and felt kind of cold "over there." He exclaimed, "Oh, no," and maneuvered two mirrors in order to see what was happening. Sure enough, what used to look like the great forests of Canada began to take on the appearance of Kansas plains. But he dismissed any thoughts of baldness. His assurance came from the fact that his father, who is at least thirty years older, had a head of hair so thick that he broke combs with it. (Even if Mike knew then that the inherited propensity was more likely from his Mom, there would not have been any clues.)

Eventually he heard comments. "Hey, Baldy, your hair is thinning out." This came as a blow, despite the harbinger years before of the cold pillow. A rigorous program of massage got under way, and he surveyed the market for help. Mike found himself wearing hats more often, not only as a cover-up (although this was a major reason), but also because hair does serve as a "fur coat." When lacking hair, one's head is indeed colder.

Soon Mike began to joke about his own bare scalp. He never considered a "rug" because a barber plopped one down on him one day, and it itched so much that he said, "Get this damn thing off before I kill it."

Mike does not anticipate that research in alopecia will advance enough to benefit him in his lifetime. But he finds that the older he gets, the easier it is to deal with his lack of hair. George Bernard Shaw has said, "Beauty is all very well at first sight; but who ever looks at it when it has been in the house three days?"[57] Mike rationalizes that the same must be true of the reverse. No one really cares about his bald head. He never tried to hide the bare spots by combing what hair he did have over the sparse areas. Yul Brynner and Kojak have helped his "macho" image. He is empathic, however, when he meets other young men who are troubled with the problem.

Mike hopes the biochemistry will be understood eventually—enough to prevent future hair loss. He is convinced it is in some way nutrition related. Heredity is strong, but he knows it can be intercepted.

If asked, Mike will tell you that he is totally adjusted to his almost bald head. In spite of his attitude, he finds himself wondering whether he should take his cap off during morning runs at the track before or after he asks Lovely Lady if she is free to have dinner with him next week-end.

MEG'S MIRROR ON THE WALL

Out, Out, Damned Spot

"To be born a woman is to know—although they do not talk of it at school—that we must labor to be beautiful."[58] It has been said that a woman cannot walk past a mirror without looking into it. In fact, it has been said for a very long time. In Shakespeare's words, "There was never yet fair woman but she made mouths in a glass."[59] Meg smiled as she caught her image. She knew at last that she would have clear skin forevermore!

Meg scrounged around in the medicine cabinet for a new tube of toothpaste, and wondered which was the most impossible dream—a

perfect man or a perfectly organized medicine cabinet. The jumbled
mess included:

> Sunburn lotion
> Rose Clay Natural deodorant
> Hair spray
> Nail polish (4 bottles)
> Nail polish remover
> Dental floss
> Perfume (many bottles)
> Eyecup
> Cotton swabs
> Toenail scissors
> Cuticle scissors
> Saline solution
> Bactine
> Tweezer
> Razor
> Baby powder
> Lipsticks, rouge, foundation creams, eye shadows, eye liners,
>   mascara, eyebrow pencils
> Diaphragm

In a far corner, some of it untouched for ten or more years:

> Nasal spray
> Eye drops
> Anesthetic medication
> Sensodyne (used once during a toothache trauma)
> Cough suppressant
> Ipecac (to induce vomiting)
> Vaseline petroleum jelly

Meg recently discarded fifteen containers of acne "cures." Despite
their absence, the medicine cabinet was still in a state of chaos.

There are few human things to which so much license, indulg-
ence, and special privilege are granted as to beauty. Meg has a superb
figure, and the grace to go with it. In her view, her Achilles' heel
stood out like a sore thumb and was on her face—in the form of blem-
ishes. But that was all in the remote past. It's been three months since
anything popped out to change the natural topography of her countenance. Meg felt as though she possessed the most coveted secret of all

time. And it was not a general practitioner, or a dermatologist, or an allergist, or an endocrinologist, or an internist, or a psychiatrist, or a gynecologist who played the ace. It was a new breed of therapist: a nutritionist.

When Meg first met with the nutrition counselor, she was promised a rose garden. The therapist was positive and enthusiastic, ready to sign in blood the fact that Meg's face would clear. Nor would Meg have to sell her soul to accomplish the goal. She would, however, have to deal with some thorns on the rose bushes. "Thorns can hurt," warned the nutritionist. "But, as with roses, the reward is more than worth the scratches." Meg was in gear, ready to accelerate at the gun, bent upon success.

Dancers who begin their careers prior to menarche (the beginning of menstruation), usually delay its onset. This is probably related to their leanness, as compared with their fatter, earlier maturing classmates.[60] Since acne and the hormones that flow so freely during puberty are interrelated, it is theorized that dancing young ladies have peaches-and-cream complexions because of the delayed puberty. But Meg did not start getting on her toes until she was sixteen, almost late for a dancer. She and acne had long since established enemy camps.

Meg's parents had been influenced by pronouncements that acne and diet have no alliance. While the traditional, or more orthodox, dermatologists were discouraging patients from changing their eating habits, the nutrition aware counselors were chalking up success after success. Recently, the *Archives of Dermatology* voiced its opinion in an editorial entitled, "Acne Diet Reconsidered," which proposed that the dermatologists have been mistaken. The researchers document the idea that hormone-dependent disease may indeed be prompted by diet.[61]

The nutrition therapist explained that acne is still the number one cause of visits to dermatologists.

Although Meg does not take any drugs, she was told about the ◻**drug**◻/acne/rash connection. Dilantin, an antiseizure medication, widely prescribed, causes skin breakouts. Antihypertensive drugs, which make people photosensitive, may be a problem. Iodides used for asthma are suspect. Lithium can cause mega acne, the cystic kind. Cortisone makes acne worse.

"Do you eat ice cream and/or milk?" Meg was asked.

"Of course."

"There are two ingredients in ice cream that may provoke skin problems. Agar, used to thicken ice cream, is a high-iodide substance. Dairy products, such as milk (also used in ice cream), may have antibiotic residues from animal feed. People allergic to penicillin may respond to milk with a rash."[62]

The Clear-Skin Diet

The wise counselor used Aristotle's philosophy: To avoid resistance and get attention, first you give before you take away. Here's the regimen:

The Additions

Good Guy Bacteria. Beauty is not only skin-deep, but its status may be traced to the innermost depths of one's body. The biochemical ecology of the intestines is as important for skin health as any topical application.

The flora of the intestinal environment is influenced by substances ingested. (Flora? Do we have plants growing inside of us? Is this the rose garden I was promised?) Intestinal flora refers to the ☆**friendly bacteria**☆ normally residing in the intestines. And yes, bacteria are classified as belonging to the plant kingdom. They are so small that angels would hardly notice the crowd if a million bacteria were sharing their space on the head of a single pin.

Some bacteria are in the service business: they help in the breakdown of dead tissue; they assist in the conversion of compounds into food; they even accommodate as a source of antibiotics.[63] User-friendly is not the exclusive domain of computers. For all these reasons, and no doubt for some we don't understand, these friendly bacteria engender skin health.

Adding small quantities of ☆**cultured milk**☆ products to the diet helps create an ideal milieu in the intestines. Three kinds of cultured milk products are easily available:

1. *Lactobacillus bulgaricus.* This is generally found in yogurt. However, if the yogurt is not homemade or not produced with carefully controlled nutritional standards, the chances are that the quantity of viable bacteria is sadly diminished, if present at all. Very few commercial brands of yogurt meet the expectations of the intestinal ambience in its quest for live, friendly bacteria.

2. *Lactobacillus acidophilus.* Acidophilus is a cultured milk product, just as yogurt is a cultured milk product. The difference is the bacteria strain. Clinical work that we have done at the Stress Center in Huntington, New York, has shown that capsules of acidophilus are not as effective as liquid acidophilus.[64] The prescription is: two tablespoons of any plain liquid acidophilus (available at natural food stores) after every meal.

3. *Lactobacillus bifidus.* Worldwide research has shown this to be the most important of the friendly intestinal flora. More bifidobacteria are found in healthy people and in mother's milk than any other variety of bacteria.[65] (Mother's milk is, after all, the only food which we know for certain is meant for human consumption.)

The biochemical ecology of the intestine is very important for the development of bifidus flora, and is most effectively influenced by human milk.[66] No, it does not mean that we should be suckling at Mother's breasts into adulthood. But there is a substance sold which is expressed from mother's milk. *Eugalan Forte* is imported from Germany, sold at natural food stores in powder form, loaded with bifidobacteria, and is a superb way of helping the intestines increase its troops of friendly soldiers.

Eastern cultures have added small amounts of fermented foods to every meal, a custom dictated by the wisdom of the ages. Because fermented foods also aid in general nutrient assimilation and digestion, it is in the best health interest of *everyone* to add a ☆**cultured product**☆ to the daily diet.

Avocados. In both animals and humans the most obvious signs of essential fatty acid deficiency are seen in the skin. When this deficiency exists, the following occurs:

1. The size of the sebaceous glands increases. Again, these are the oil-secreting glands under the skin, which secrete sebum.
2. Sebum production increases. Sebum is a thick, semifluid, greasy, lubricating substance composed of fat and epithelial (skin) debris.[67] The sebum is carried to the outer edges of the skin by ducts, and excreted from the skin through openings, or pores.

Essential fatty acids are available in supplemental form. Cod-liver oil and gamma linolenic acid are examples. Meg's wise counselor, however, does not want to perpetuate the myth of the magic bullet.

A single nutrient, pill, tablet, capsule, or tablespoon of a product is not enough to promote good health. If a healthful food which contains important nutrients is included in the diet, the ratio of good and bad foods must begin to change. Once this concept is understood and practiced, the nutrition counselor recommends the use of supplements (especially those with gamma linolenic acid) for recalcitrant skin conditions.

Avocados are an excellent food rich in essential fatty acids. Meg adds a quarter of an avocado to her lunch salad every day, and rubs the inside of the peel on her skin. (She answered her doorbell one day, confused when her visitor stared at her and said, "Are the Martians here?" She forgot she had a green face!) Topical application of essential fatty acids is also beneficial.

Cold-water ☆**fish**☆ such as cod, salmon, mackerel, halibut, sea bass, and weakfish also contain essential fatty acids. Meg was advised to include cold-water fish three times a week, and to eat the skin of the fish.

Fiber. A large salad of *raw* ☆**vegetables**☆ is part of the daily regimen. The salad must be comprised of at least six or seven different varieties of vegetables, including one grated carrot. In addition, a pot of lightly steamed vegetables—again, consisting of an assortment—must be consumed every day. Aside from the ☆**vitamin**☆ and ☆**mineral**☆ content, vegetables assist digestion and elimination.

It didn't take long for Meg to appreciate the fact that lettuce, tomatoes, and cucumbers do not a salad made, or that overcooked ▫**canned**▫ or ▫**frozen**▫ peas and carrots are low on the totem pole for skin health. She thoroughly enjoyed the heterogeneity of the salad and vegetable platters, which presented new taste treats.

To solve the problem of dinner invitations, Meg always offers to bring the salad. This gives her assurance that at least part of the meal will be healthful. Her friends welcome the offering, describing the preparation as containing everything but the kitchen sink. Meg responded by buying a dollhouse-sized kitchen sink, which she places atop her salads. The salads have come to be known as "Meg's Kitchen Sink Salads."

Vitamin A foods. The "turnover" rate of skin cells is about twenty-eight days. Since ☆**vitamin A**☆ is essential for new cell growth, it provides one of the most important aspects of metabolic functions in the maintenance of normal epithelium.[68] Vitamin A is concentrated only in certain tissues of animal products in which the animal has metabolized the carotene contained in its food into vitamin A. Fish-liver oil is the richest source of vitamin A.

Carotene, which the body converts into vitamin A, is found in carrots (from which its name is derived), beet greens, spinach, broccoli, and any other ☆vegetable☆ of bright orange, red, or yellow color. ☆**Green leafy vegetables**☆ contain more usable carotene than carrots do! In addition to the raw and lightly steamed platters already outlined, Meg includes cantaloupes and peaches.

Preparations of pure beta-carotene are on the market, but once again, the counselor prefers real food as a source of vitamin A—at least until Meg fully understands the concept.

Progesterone and Sulfur. No, not in pill form, but progesterone is a fabulous skin nutrient. It is produced in the body when vitamin A and niacin are present, and these nutrients are found in ☆**liver**☆ ☆**eggs**☆, and sweet potatoes. Since the sulfur in eggs tends to shrink and reduce inflammation of pimples, egg on your face is not a bad idea after all. Another trick is to use beaten egg whites to tighten the skin.[69]

Supplements. As stated, the therapist initiates food changes first. When it is evident that the patient is complying, the following recommendations are made:

> ☆**Vitamin C**☆, to prevent acne infection
> ☆**Vitamin B$_6$**☆, to reduce facial oiliness
> ☆**Vitamin A**☆, to heal and clear skin
> ☆**Vitamin E**☆, applied topically, to avoid acne scars [70]
> ☆**gamma linolenic acid**☆, to supply the PUFAs

The Subtractions

The Wrong Kind of Fatty Foods. The same enzyme systems handle similar fats in the body. Nonessential fatty acids are those which the body can manufacture. They do not have to come from the food you eat. Essential fatty acids must be in the food supply. Large amounts of nonessential saturated fatty acids compete with essential fatty acids and suppress their activity. This internal civil war results in a reduction of essential fatty acids. To avoid the problem, avoid the enemy: eliminate or cut down on foods containing nonessential, □**processed**□ saturated fats, such as modern-day meat, processed cheese, ersatz ice cream products, nondairy coffee creamers, bakery products, potato chips, crackers, mixes, and so on.

Intensification of animal management has resulted both in an increase in the amount of saturated fat and a reduction in the amount of essential fatty acids per unit of meat eaten. This is caused by restriction of exercise in domestic animals, use of high energy foods to feed these animals, and genetic selection for the fast-growing animal. The increase of adipose fat leads to intramuscular infiltration of triglycerides, known as "marbling" in the livestock industry. These triglycerides are mainly composed of nonessential saturated fatty acids, and their deposit further increases the amount of saturated fats and also reduces the nutrient value per unit of meat weight.[71] In light of these facts, an additional recommendation is to eat very little meat, if any.

Acid Foods. Crucial advice is to eliminate the following foods: citrus fruit, coffee, tomatoes, soda, pineapple, milk, nuts, and corn. One more limitation: *no salt.*

The Exercise Connection

Meg was told that people with acne have lower levels of high-density lipoproteins. (Remember? Those are the good guy portions of cholesterol.) The meaning of this finding with respect to skin problems remains to be studied.[72] Since aerobic exercise increases high-density lipoproteins, Meg knew she was on track by being on the track!

Meg questioned the nutrition counselor concerning the new retinoids used in dermatology. They are synthetically developed vitamin A derivatives, extraordinarily effective in controlling a wide variety of skin diseases. The answer is twofold:

(1) Unhealthy skin is a symptom, not a disease. If the symptom is suppressed, the cause may never be corrected. When retinoid therapy is stopped, there are relapses.[73]

(2) Many adverse reports are flooding the medical literature. One indicates skeletal toxicity with long-term administration of retinoic acid.[74,75] Other complaints are nosebleeds, conjunctivitis, and a dry rash elsewhere on the body.[76] The retinoids work because of their toxicity.

Meg inquired about a regimen for atopic eczema, a condition suffered by a close friend. She and her friend often commiserated about their complexions. The counselor advised that gamma linolenic acid produces improvement in many people.[77] Sounding like a broken record, the counselor offered the same advice for oily skin, dry skin, flaky skin, acne, atopic eczema, or even psoriasis.

As a matter of fact, this regimen is also preventive. If you've never had a blemish, but want the best insurance against wrinkles, the best insurance against dried-out aging skin, the best insurance for the best complexion, *this program is for you.*

For the first time in her life, Meg did not feel the need for applications of makeup. She wondered if Fellow with Blue Cap had noticed the difference. "He should—he certainly looks at me closely enough each day."

"Loveliness needs not the foreign aid of ornament. But is, when unadorned, adorned the most."[78]

SALLY'S SALVATION

Move Your Stuff Over, Tom

"What a mess I am! Jaw sagging; skin flabby; neck full of wrinkles; bags under my eyes; hair thinning. Too bad my eyesight's so perfect."

Sally recalled the reaction she and Tom had when they looked at their daughter's wedding proofs just the other day. She said, "I look fat in these pictures." Tom said, "I look old." They did not say, "I *am* fat," or "I *am* old." The inference? The photographer was at fault. "The photographer won't be able to squeeze us into standard formats," teased Sally. "Maybe we should order 14 × 14s, instead of 8 × 10s." Tom, with his usual twinkle added, "Do you think they print 1 × 12s for Twiggy?"

Sally started to freshen up, which in her case, she said, could take a week. She knew she was not aging gracefully. Aristotle said, "Personal beauty is a greater recommendation than any letter of reference."[79] This sentiment has been echoed by every generation since Aristotle. It is one of the facts of life that plain people like Sally have to put up with. But since she started her exercise program, she had a plan. She was waiting for the propitious moment before sharing her idea with Tom.

Tom! That hypochondriac! Look at all this stuff sitting in this medicine chest:

Product for fever blisters (judging from the low price tag which
 was still firmly affixed, it had to be at least 20 years old)
Product for cold sores
Demerol Hydro Chloride, which is actually dope and may even be
 illegal
Instant shoe coloring (why is shoe polish in the medicine cabi-
 net?)
Mycolog cream (for the dog?)
Hydrogen peroxide
Iodine
Cheracol
Ichthammol ointment
Antacids
Peptobismol
Lomotil
Gelusil
Auralgin
Mylanta
Bandages, regular
Bandages, butterfly
Antibiotic ointment
Benzocaine
Suppositories
Fleet enema kits
After-shave medicated cream
Cleacinan acid to remove warts
Calamine lotion
Orinase for diabetes
Digitalis
Benedryl
K-tabs
Tenormin
Hydrochlorothiazide
Nicobid
Tolinase

Tom was ready for anything short of an appendectomy. (Maybe that too: several small scalpels and a pair of scissors were concealed in the recesses of these narrow shelves.)

If Tom felt comfortable having this small hospital on hand, no matter. What did concern Sally was that it limited *her* space for products she considered more vital:

Scalp and hair conditioner (it doesn't say what condition it leaves you with)
Skin clearer (expiration date, 1963)
Nail satin
Soft luster for skin
Suntan lotion
Gillette lady's razor
Complete makeup for flawless, radiant beauty
No-peroxide color lotion to wash away gray
Liquid rouge
Dandruff shampoos
A piece of soap from a hotel in Costa Rica
A free sample of something that looks like toilet paper for a guinea pig
A piece of soap from KLM, with a Spanish name

Tom had minor difficulties (a little bit of diabetes, a little bit of heart trouble, a little bit of high triglycerides, and so on). Sally and the children continued to tease him about focusing too much attention on his health. Tom good-naturedly accepted the family's jokes, and responded with a few himself.

Tom: "I may look healthy, but under all this tan, you should know how pale I am."

Sally: "The way you feel, can I take a chance and buy you a five-year calendar?"

Tom: "I'm so full of medicine, every time I sneeze, I cure somebody."

Their daughter: "My father's such a hypochondriac, he won't even talk to me on the phone if I have a cold."

Tom: "You people are such sadists. You're not supposed to tell a hypochondriac how well he looks, or send me 'get well' cards. Besides, I hope I'm sick. I'd hate to be well and feel like this."

Sally: "Tom won't let 'well enough' alone."

Sally's plan evolved slowly. Despite her lack of beauty, she had a good self-image. She was bright, capable, and happy, and accepted the fact that all women over 45 begin to experience very specific changes. She read:

Skinfold measurements indicate [that the thinning of the outermost layers of skin] begins with regularity at age 45. . . . Other constituents of the skin undergo regression, including the elastic fibers in the subcutaneous layer and sweat glands, which also diminish in number. The net effect leaves the skin in a dry, thin, inelastic state. . . . The skin of Caucasians tends to become more pallid; this is sometimes further accentuated by the loss of ruddiness because of decreased peripheral circulation in the small blood vessels. Deposits of pigmentation are also seen (melanotic freckles), although the skin overall seems paler. In addition, brown plaquelike growths (seborrheic hyperkatoses) the size of a small coin appear more and more after age 50. . . . Wrinkling or permanent infoldings of the skin, a result of skin sagging and loss of elasticity, are most often noted on the face because of repeated stress on facial skin produced by the muscles of expression. Wrinkling is more severe in those exposed to the sun. The neck is perhaps the most reliable area in which to observe aging change, usually quite obvious by age 50. Other common sites are above the eyebrows and at the outer edges of the lips and mouth. By age 50, the lobes of the ear become fuller, and the ear seems more elongated.[80]

One need only to study a child's face to see the aging process in reverse: larger eyes, shorter nose, smooth skin, and fuller cheeks.

Sally knows that multiple factors, such as heredity, diet, □stress□, sex, and environmental conditions play a role in the aging process. Not everyone is going to lose elasticity or develop saggy-baggy eyelids on the day of his or her forty-fifth birthday. Could Sally have delayed the process if she had awakened to the benefits of nutrition and exercise at an earlier age? Actually, every time she sought a nutritional remedy for a problem it seemed to work. For example:

- When she recognized that she was developing body odor, she read about the use of ☆**magnesium**☆ and ☆**zinc**☆, along with vitamins ☆**B₆**☆ and ☆**PABA**☆ (para-aminobenzoic acid). The report stated that this was effective, not only for offensive body odors, but also for breath odors. It is theorized that the nutrients act as waste scavengers, removing substances that give off acrid odors in the body.[81] The skin is a major detoxifying organ. Many volatile gasses are discharged through it, so that sharp body odors can be an indication of poor nutrient balance.[82]
- When Sally developed both a small lump and sagging breasts, she investigated estrogen treatment, learning that it is not very good for restoring firmness, and can be risky—especially if a lump is present.[83] Eliminating □**coffee**□ (not an easy task) was the effective therapy for getting rid of the lump.[84]

- Years back, when Sally suffered from premenstrual syndrome (which may be average, but is not normal), she used a nutritional approach to relieve the depression, irritability, edema, cramps, headache, and mood swings which surfaced each month. The program consisted of several grams of ☆vitamin C☆, ☆vitamin A☆, ☆B₆☆, ☆folic acid☆, and ☆gamma linolenic acid☆. After a couple of months, it worked.[85]
- Every now and then Sally developed cracks in the corners of her mouth. One doctor suggested the possibility of herpes, another asked her if she had vacationed in a dry climate, or if she had gone skiing in a very cold vacation spot. A friend suggested lack of niacin and/or riboflavin, labeling the problem cheilosis. The ☆B complex☆ did the trick.[86]

With the exception of the handful of nutrition tricks, the only other attempt Sally made to improve her appearance was the use of a padded bra. The joke between Tom and herself was that she violated the "truth in packaging" law.

"Well," thought Sally, "maybe I missed the boat until recently, but I know now. Yes, I'm going to do it. I just have to figure out when to tell Tom."

Sally was inspired by an interview she heard. Dr. Joseph Consentino, renowned plastic surgeon of New York, said:

Those of us who are distressed about the contemplation of age should become thrilled at the thought that we have this prospect facing us, for the alternative concerns us not.

Of course as we age there is an absorption of subcutaneous fat and interstitial tissue, which accounts for a good deal of our changing body and skin surface. The end result is a loosening of skin, particularly around exposed parts of the body. The nose appears longer, the skin around the eyelids, chin, face, and neck plus other areas becomes redundant. We do know also that the bony structure of the entire skeletal system goes through a process of shrinking, adding to the obvious appearance of aging.

When this point has been reached, not only is cosmetic intervention for restoration of a youthful expression or appearance something to consider, but primarily a review of the proper diet is of utmost importance.

Major aging factors are □smoking□ and □sun□ exposure. The parts of the body which age more quickly are those that are not covered, and which have fewer oil glands.

It would be unusual for someone *not* to want to feel younger and look younger.[87]

Dr. Consentino's interview convinced Sally that people who *feel* that they look good, feel better about themselves. The most common reasons for cosmetic surgery are marital difficulties, little success at home or on the job, and a desire to recapture lost beauty. Women age more readily than men. A man can tolerate the sun better because his beard acts as many little poles in the skin, supporting and smoothing it. Not that it's a cover-up: the practice of shaving causes the removal of some of the fine superficial wrinkles every morning.

The Pre-Op Program

Sally was convinced that better nutrition and life-style could have slowed the aging process. The adjustments she was making by reducing indiscretions (she was ☆**exercising**☆, not ▫smoking▫, and consuming more ☆**healthful food products**☆), would, she hoped, allow her to grow old gracefully. The surgery would erase a few past mistakes. Once Sally made the decision to have the minor plastic surgery, she was elated. "You never get a second chance to make a good first impression."

In addition to getting rid of fatty folds on her eyelids, all those "beauty" marks on her face would be removed. She was told that she could anticipate both friends and relatives saying, "Gee, you look terrific. Have you been away?" or, "Have you changed your hair style?" Perfect! The surgery would not be noticed. The aim of aesthetic surgery is to create a natural appearance. Just the change Sally needed. A permanent "retouching" of her baggy eyes and her not-so-smooth skin. How exciting!

Tom was in the midst of an involved business transaction. Sally decided it was wise to wait until his dealings were resolved before discussing her desire for the surgery. Tom always appeared anxious during these long decision-making trials with his associates. Yet he was such a good businessman, Sally was convinced he could sell American transistor radios in Japan! In any case, she did not want to add to his stress at this time. Somehow she anticipated that he would voice objections.

Meanwhile, Sally gathered information about pre- and postoperative priming, detailed by Dr. Howard Bezoza, nutrition oriented surgeon of New York City:

- No ▫smoking▫ or ▫coffee▫ for two weeks before surgery. This is to (1) avoid withdrawal from these drugs during surgery, and (2) encourage good blood vessel flow. Both nicotine and caffeine cause vasoconstriction, which in turn diminishes oxygen that would be brought to the area of surgery.

- Start simple breathing exercises two weeks before surgery to increase oxygenation. Taking ☆**long walks**☆ may be the easiest way to accomplish this goal.
- Drink lots of ☆**water**☆. As estrogen diminishes, the ability to maintain hydration becomes somewhat impaired. This is one of the reasons why the skin becomes a little more raggedy and wrinkly. A minimum of six glasses a day is necessary.
- The important nutrients in wound healing are:

  (a) ☆**Zinc**☆—the definitive cofactor for the ability to cross-link collagen; in other words, to hold it together. Collagen is the main supportive protein of skin, tendon, bone, cartilage, and connective tissue. It represents approximately 30 percent of total body protein.

  (b) ☆**Ascorbic acid**☆—the nutrient that plays a critical role in wound repair as a cofactor during collagen manufacture.

  (c) ☆**Sulphur**☆—sulphur amino acids are necessary in cross-bonding. [☆**Eggs**☆ contain sulphur amino acids.]

- If available, get involved in sauna or whirlpool therapy. Sitting in a steam room and getting massages provides muscular relaxation, and increases the amount of blood flow without muscle use. This, like exercise, helps in the removal of cellular waste products. The ancients gathered in the baths, not so much to be social, but mainly because it made them feel better—they were oxygenating their tissues.
- Following surgery, ☆**vitamin E**☆ may be used as a topical agent. It is an antioxidant, which means it prevents bacterial growth. It helps stabilize the membranes of cells, thereby decreasing the incidence of wound breakdown. This helps override excessive scarring.
- Instead of □codeine□, which is constipating, the aloe vera plant should be used as a superior anesthetic. It may prove to be the best local anesthetic around. [Imagine that statement made by an American surgeon?] Since pure aloe vera is not easy to secure, the best alternative is to buy the plant itself. If it weren't for aloe vera, South American Indians and native American Indians would probably not have survived in the sun. These groups were not dark-complected, and therefore did not have protecting pigment.[88,89]

Sally Tells Tom

The day finally came. Tom and his business associates signed their contract. Sally revealed her desire to Tom. She had anticipated Benjamin Franklin's attitude: "Beauty and folly are old companions."[90] Instead, his response astounded her. He not only supported her decision, but added, "I really need it more than you do. Look at these folds under my eyes. Every time I meet with young executives, I feel older and older."

Sally shared her pre-op nutrition information with Tom. He wanted to start the nutrition regimen at once, weeks before they could even make an appointment to see the plastic surgeon. "Tom," said Sally, "it's only a minor operation. No great amount of blood is lost." Tom answered, "A minor operation is an operation performed on somebody else. We'd better start getting ready now."

Sally could hardly wait for her new look. She felt it was just the "lift" she needed to inspire her to go places—other than from home to the store. She knew that her improved appearance would not solve any problems or improve any performance. Sally had no unrealistic expectations. She watched Leo Buscaglia on Phil Donahue's program, and heard his message: "Nothing is enough until *you* are enough." Sally sensed that she required the minor change in order to help her feel that *she* was enough.

JIM AND JANE AND CHANGING APOTHECARIES

Gone: The Dandruff Dilemma

Jane and Jim no longer kept aspirin on hand. They had learned the headache secret: Six ☆calcium☆ tablets and some ☆B complex☆—the magic formula. They're happy to say that they rarely get headaches any more. But should a headache sneak in, the calcium and the B complex do the trick.

Remnants of their old life-style, however, still vie for space on the narrow shelves of their medicine cabinet:

> Baby powder
> Acne medicine, superstrength
> Antihistamine
> Cough syrup

Campho-phenique pain reliever
Prescription drug for chest congestion
Neosynephrine nose drops
Auralgan for earaches

As a consequence of their new consciousness, these items began to replace more traditional medical and beauty supports:

☆**Herbal**☆ shampoo
Organic hair treatment
Clay face mask
Neem toothpaste, derived from the bark of a tree
☆**Brewer's yeast**☆ skin cream
Aloe vera burn relief cream
Homeopathic cold remedy
☆**Vitamin E**☆ capsules for topical application
☆**Herbal**☆ foot lotion
Apple cider vinegar (for final hair rinse)

With great ceremony, Jane and Jim have already discarded their old dandruff preparations, along with other commercial hair concoctions. Dr. Irwin Lubowe, known for his work in promoting healthy hair, states that the basic causes of dandruff are a faulty diet, emotional tension, hormonal disturbance, infection due to disease, injury to the scalp, and unwise or excessive use of hair cosmetics.[91] Jane and Jim's armamentarium of "looking-good-tips" for hair includes this information:

- Dr. John Yudkin of England believes that a high sugar intake can be a major contributing cause of dandruff.[92] Since dandruff is a mild form of seborrheic dermatitis, and ☆**B complex**☆ components are an antidote for this condition, the sugar theory makes sense. Sugar requires B vitamins in order to be metabolized. Too much sugar exhausts the B vitamin supply, leaving none to counter the scalp condition.
- When the bloodstream provides the hair with plenty of proteins, fats, carbohydrates, ☆**enzymes**☆, and ☆**minerals**☆, hair flourishes. If these nutrients are in short supply, the hair is undernourished.[93]
- Acne-enhancing foods also promote dandruff, because they encourage sebum production. The culprits are: chocolate, nuts, shellfish, iodized salt, butter, □**fried foods**□, and □**alcohol**□.[94]
- Hair sprays, permanent wave lotions, bleaches, cosmetics, and de-

tergent shampoos can also lead to dandruff through their scaling and drying actions.[95]

- Grandma may have been right about garlic, eating for two during pregnancy, cod-liver oil, and other wonderful folk practices, but she missed the boat when she recommended one hundred hairbrush strokes a day. Too much brushing is not good for your scalp or your hair's appearance.

The following processes and products should be used moderately, if totally unavoidable: bleaching, teasing, roller curlers, curling wands, blow dryers, hair straighteners, hair sprays, permanent wave lotions, and electric curlers. The most prized and expensive wigs are made from hair of women who have not exposed their crowning glory to any cosmetics—ever![96]

- Jane's Mom had been complaining of losing her hair. This propelled Jane and Jim to investigate hair loss in women, a problem occurring with increasing frequency. Dr. Howard Bezoza points out that female hair loss is related to several hormonal functions, to vascular problems, to nutrient levels (or the body's inability to deliver the nutrients to the hair), and also to what women have been doing to their hair.

Sometimes it's "Catch-22." The more sparse the hair becomes, the harder it is to manage, and the more improper handling may be employed. Measures that may make the coiffure more attractive, but increase the amount of hair loss, are intensified, such as the use of hot driers and curlers.

Dr. Bezoza explains that although the thyroid continues to function as we get older, the tissues of the body lose their capacity to absorb thyroid hormones. This causes a reduced elasticity of capillaries, resulting in loss of nutrients to tissue—including scalp tissue. ☆**Vitamin C**☆ and ☆zinc☆ are nutrients which help maintain capillary function.[97] Dr. Carl Pfeiffer states that some of the best results in hair strength and restoration have occurred when patients get adequate zinc, vitamin B_6, and ☆**egg**☆ yolks. The egg yolks are an excellent source of sulfur-containing nutrients.[98]

Since hair loss may be precipitated by excessive dandruff, the same regimen outlined for that problem would be helpful. To stimulate circulation, which is essential for the delivery of nutrients to hair follicles, gentle massaging of the scalp is also suggested.

▫**Processed**▫ foods are nutrient depleted. A diet of ☆**whole natural foods**☆ is the best insurance for avoiding hair loss problems, for arresting its continued progress if it already exists, and may even be helpful in *reversing* damage done.

Listening to her parents discuss hair overhaulings (no more dandruff, shinier and silkier hair, Grandma's sparse hair, and so on), inspired eight-year-old Janie to recite a nonsense verse she had learned:

> I'd rather have fingers than toes,
> I'd rather have eyes than a nose;
> And as for my hair
> I'm glad it's all there,
> I'll be awfully sad when it goes.[99]

KEITH AND TEETH AND MORE

Covering the Gray

Pasted on the mirror of Keith's medicine cabinet was another mirror—a small, circular magnifying glass. Every morning Keith examined his teeth closely. Was the Topol working? Topol was his ammunition to eradicate the stains on his teeth.

Lodged within the cupboard behind the mirrors:

> Grecian Formula
> Saline solution (for contact lenses)
> Daily cleanser (for contact lenses)
> Enzymatic (for contact lenses)
> Phenobarbital (not used recently)
> Skin cream
> Antiperspirants
> Compound for drying runny noses
> Solarcane
> Lotion for dry skin
> Nasal spray
> Matches (to annihilate bathroom odors)
> Baby powder
> Visine
> Soothing eye lotion
> Cough suppressant

Corn remover
Hair-grooming products
Touch-up (blemish cover-up)
Toothpaste for sensitive teeth
Porcelain coating to cover veins
Medicine for diarrhea
Throat lozenges
Mouth rinses

Keith is handsome and vain. His most prominent aging marker is kept under control with hair dyes. An exposé of these dyes informed Keith that most of them are not harmless.

Natural hair dyes (such as henna, which is a vegetable dye) have been used for many hundreds, if not thousands, of years. They are not as popular as the commercial preparations because they are not as consistent or easy to use. But they are also not injurious.

Lead, silver, and copper have been applied to conceal gray hair since the days of ancient Rome, and are still in use. These metallic dyes should not be used by women who have permanents because there is a lack of compatibility between the metals and waving solutions. Men, however, do resort to formulas containing lead, in spite of the fact that lead is a suspected carcinogen.

□Coal-tar dyes□ used in hair-coloring products are also hazardous. Researchers have correlated these dyes with leukemia and mutagenic effects. The General Accounting Office Survey of Cosmetics, presented to Congress in the late 1970s, revealed that more than one hundred ingredients used in cosmetics are suspected of causing cancer. Many hair-coloring products are among those indicted.[100]

This knowledge has been no deterrent for Keith. But he is willing to try another route. If it works, he will give up the dyes. Since ☆pantothenic acid☆ deficiency promotes gray hair, Keith is hopeful that its use might restore natural color. ☆Zinc☆ and sulphur have also been reported to reverse the graying process.[101] Other studies herald ☆PABA☆ (para-aminobenzoic acid) as the panacea. Keith is trying them all.

In addition to taking these substances in supplement form, Keith is beginning to gain knowledge about *why* these nutrients have been in short supply in his diet. Pantothenic acid, for example, is required in greater quantities after any kind of injury, after antibiotic therapy, or during the stress of any severe illness.[102] Pantothenic acid is widely distributed in foods, but only in very low concentrations. Although it abounds, there is not much of it in any single food product.

In a recent study, 597 edible products were analyzed for pantothenic acid content. Losses of this nutrient due to processing are very significant:

Pantothenic Acid Losses

◻Canned◻ foods, animal origin	losses up to 35%
◻Canned◻ foods, vegetable origin	losses up to 78%
◻Frozen◻ foods, animal origin	losses up to 70%
◻Frozen◻ foods, vegetable origin	losses up to 57%
◻Canned◻ fruit & fruit juices	losses up to 50%
◻Refined◻ grains (white flour, etc.)	losses up to 74%
◻Processed◻ meats	losses up to 75% [103]

No studies have been done to determine antagonistic effects of ◻drugs◻, ◻pollutants◻, or other environmental indiscretions upon the metabolism of pantothenic acid, which would probably increase the percentage of losses. Since there is not much pantothenic acid in any one food product to begin with, it is obvious that anyone not consuming foods in their natural, unprocessed state runs the risk of deficiency. If people are becoming gray earlier on, it is no wonder.

The ◻Nicotine◻ Smile

Keith never took the time to question how or why his tooth stain remover works. If he looked at the label, this would not be much help, unless he knew that silicate is an abrasive, contained in building materials such as cement, concrete, bricks, and glass.

Keith is certain that his self-administration of nicotine will soon be a habit of the past. He hopes the cues that trigger "lighting up" will diminish. The stimulant he expects to take over and have full command? Running. One of his friends predicted that he will be the worst reformed smoker ever—in terms of being critical of other smokers. He already chastised his brother-in-law for puffing away in his sister's face, citing that passive smoking takes four years off a nonsmoking woman's life.[104] There is also a significantly increased risk of lung cancer in nonsmoking women if their husbands smoke.[105] But so far it's all talk. Keith is still puffing away.

Vanity is why Keith rates nicotine stains as his number one dental problem. His dentist, however, considers his gum problems of a more serious nature. Fortunately, his dentist is among those who recognize the relationship between periodontal disease and nutrients. The dentist has explained that periodontal tissue (the connective tissue interposed between the teeth and their bony sockets) is susceptible to inflammation and degeneration in the presence of a local irritant, whether it is a foreign body or food debris.[106] Under conditions of malnutrition, the bone withdrawal and inflammation are intensified. Protein deficiency in particular impairs the strength of the tissues surrounding the inflamed area and slows down the rate of healing.[107]

On the basis of our present knowledge, deficiencies of ☆**protein**☆, ☆**ascorbic acid**☆, ☆**B complex**☆ vitamins, ☆**vitamin A**☆, and ☆**mineralizing**☆ nutrients such as ☆**calcium**☆, phosphorus, and ☆**vitamin D**☆, may adversely condition the health of the periodontium—important tissues supporting the teeth.[108]

Gingiva, or mucous membrane, with its fibrous tissue, encircles the necks of teeth. When this gummy area of the mouth is diseased, it is said to be a manifestation of scurvy, which indicates a ☆**vitamin C**☆ deficiency. But again, a local irritation must be present before the vitamin C deficiency can produce its worsening of the gums.[109] Therefore, administration of vitamin C without attacking the precipitating mechanism may not suffice.

Experiments with calcium/phosphorus ratios reveal the importance of the balance between these two minerals. If there is too much phosphorus present, the body reabsorbs ☆**calcium**☆ from bony structures in its effort to maintain the proper ratio. There is a liberation of skeletal calcium reserves in order to raise the blood levels of calcium, which in turn balance phosphorus levels. The result is bone loss—the sacrifice of skeletal tissues. The integrity of gums and teeth is affected, among other problems. This may even be the first symptom of osteoporosis (bone disease characterized by reduction in bone density). Osteoporosis is a common occurrence in our country.

The important question is: what causes an improper balance? What causes an overabundance of phosphorus? The answer is *the average American diet!* Pick up any soft drink (diet or otherwise), and you will notice the additive "phosphoric this" or "phosphoric that" (sodium phosphate; phosphoric acid; and so on). Additional sources of phosphorus are obtained from hot dogs, ham, bacon, ▢**processed**▢ and ▢**canned**▢ meat, processed cheese, many baked products (with phosphate baking powder commonly used), instant soups and puddings, toppings and seasonings.[110] Is it any wonder that we are taxing our parathyroids, those wonderful glands whose job it is to maintain calcium and phosphorus balances?

Another aspect of good periodontal health involves ☆**fibrous foods**☆. Unfortunately, there are misconceptions. Chewing hard foods will *not* remove plaque (deposits of material on the surface of teeth, which may serve as a medium for growth of bacteria, or as a nucleus for the initiation of periodontal disease). Firm foods can, however, stimulate salivary flow and therefore can aid in the oral clearance of food debris. Chewing fibrous foods can also strengthen the periodontal ligament and increase the density of the bony structure supporting the teeth.[111,112,113]

In discussing foods that might ensure better periodontal health and reduce the incidence of cavities, Keith's dentist, tongue in cheek, offered a recipe consumed by a group of primitive people who were cavity free. The recipe: baked cod's head stuffed with oatmeal and chopped cod's ☆**livers**☆. The oats and fish, including livers, provide ☆**minerals**☆ and ☆**vitamins**☆ adequate for an excellent racial stock with high immunity to tooth decay.[114]

There is evidence to show that the progress of periodontal disease can be retarded by flossing. The procedure is to hold the floss tautly, sliding it between teeth. Then curve it into a C-shape against one tooth and gently slide it into the space between gum and tooth until resistance is met. The floss should then be moved away from the gums, while still holding it tightly against the tooth. Repeat this procedure for both sides of each tooth.

Water irrigation devices serve to flush out accumulated toxic material from under the gums, from periodontal pockets. The problem is that people expect more from these devices than they can produce. Plaque is the main cause of gingival irritation. Plaque consists of active germ colonies that grow on teeth above and below the gumline. Toxins coming from plaque debilitate the inner parts of the gum pocket. Water irrigators wash most of this foul material out, *but the irrigation will not break up the plaque that is causing the problem.*

These devices should not be used with any force. The solution pumped into the area can bruise the delicate tissues and then the toxic wastes may actually be forced into one's bloodstream.

Keith's dentist cautioned him against eating sugar with highly refined starch. (Jelly or honey on white bread would be an example.) The cavity promoting effect is worse than eating sugar alone. Sugars are, of course, the most important dietary cause of cavities. Evidence incriminating sugars continues to accumulate.[115]

When Keith jokingly asked his dentist why people get severe

toothaches on holiday week-ends, he was given information on temporary measures to relieve toothache pain. A drop or two of hot-pepper extract applied on cotton to a sore tooth was recommended in 1850 as an instant remedy for toothache. More than a century later, we understand the mechanism. The pungent principle of hot paprika or chili peppers is capsicum which selectively stimulates and then blocks the sensitive sensory nerves of the skin and mucous membranes.[116]

The chemical structure of capsicum is similar to that of eugenol, the active principle of oil of cloves, which also can induce a long-lasting local anesthesia.[117,118] Chewing on cloves from the condiment box, or on a ☆**vitamin E**☆ capsule, are two additional tricks for relieving toothache. And yet another is the application of aloe vera because of its anesthetic properties.

Keith, like so many Americans, has put more effort into correcting tooth damage than into preventing further deterioration. Many people seek caps and bridges, each spending thousands. If the same effort and money were directed toward nutrition education and behavior modification to facilitate life-style changes, would we need the dentist—except for accidents?

★   ★   ★

The camouflage cabinets are slid open and closed daily. We continue to strive for our best image projection. The commercial interests flood the market, ever in search of the ultimate in cover-up products.

Jean Kerr has said, "I'm tired of all this nonsense about beauty not being only skin-deep. What do you want—an adorable pancreas?" Well, yes, that's exactly what we want. And an elegant liver. And a springtide spleen. A youthful thyroid. A pretty pituitary. And most definitely a resplendent brain!

We should be able to leave this world young as late as possible.

CHAPTER 3

The Scale Association

Rhoda weighs two hundred and fifty pounds. She made an appointment with a diet doctor. He looked at her and said, "My, you are obese." Rhoda answered, "I want a second opinion."

"Starve her slowly."

"Pour liquid food down her throat, and nothing else."

"No, no, take out most of her intestines."

"No. Dried food. Maybe in powder form."

"Frozen food. That's it. Only frozen packets."

"Send her to the gym and make her sweat it off."

"No. She won't go. Sell her expensive home equipment."

"Not expensive. A jump rope. All day long."

"I have an idea. Put a balloon in her stomach."

"A pill. Give her the prescriptions."

"Don't bother. She has them. Illegally."

"Wrap her stomach in gauze."

"Make her read a new diet book—every day."

"Send her to a hypnotist."

"Modify her behavior."

"Put a staple in her ear."

"Wire her mouth shut."

"Elevate her mood."

"Stuff her with methyl cellulose or some other unabsorbable bulk."

"Alter the setting of her appetite regulating center in her hypothalamus."

"No, no. Stick something in her brain and kill part of it."[1]

On a recent panel discussion, an overweight lady expressed this
thought: "We can't say anything about racism. We can't say anything
about sexism. We can't say anything about any physical disability. But
one last safe prejudice still exists for Americans. It's okay to knock *fat*
because it's our fault. Well, I have a message for everyone: *it's not our
fault.*"

A fat woman was stopped in the supermarket by another shopper.
"We're starting a reducing club," she was told, "and we need about a
dozen members before we can get our franchise." "Oh," answered the
large lady, "let me think. Who do I know that's overweight? Give me
your number. If anyone comes to mind, I'll let them know about your
group." The embarrassed shopper said, "Oh, I didn't mean you. I mean
. . . I just thought . . ." She left, rather confused. Some people reluctantly accept their overweight status and use it to laugh at themselves and embarrass others.

DR. SMITH EXPLAINS "SET POINT"

Mission Impossible May Be Possible

Despite redundancy of assistance (books, pills, clubs, therapists,
gyms), endless patients stream into Dr. Bob Smith's office asking for
guidance. The questions, pleas, and comments are always the same:

"Last year I got rid of my flab. This year I have new flab."

"I'm a light eater. As soon as it gets light, I start eating."

"I need a mouth blocker, not a starch blocker."

"I'm getting so fat, I got my shoes shined and had to take the guy's
word for it."

"I haven't been able to diet in a month of sundaes."

"I'm on a seafood diet. When I see food, I eat it."

"Eating a carrot at a baseball game isn't exactly a hit."

And plain "Help!"

Bob knows there are only two ways to lose weight. One is to starve,
and we all know that doesn't work. The other is to get involved in a
regular program of aerobic exercise, and we all know that doesn't work—
well, hardly ever. Exercising has a better track record than starving,

but it requires motivation. The usual response to the "get moving" suggestion is, "I don't have time." The argument that *you get that time back because you have more energy when you exercise* is ineffectual, despite its credibility. "It's as frustrating as attempting to hold two watermelons in one hand," says Bob. (But he does try. Not the watermelons—the behavior modification.)

Bob uses many modalities in his motivation schemes. If the patient is willing to participate, either through Bob's efforts or because the patient is ready, success is around the corner. A major thrust is to dispel myths, explain set point, and discuss nutrition. Bob brings into play as many approaches as there are variations in awareness. Everyone appears to be at a different niche on the health/insight continuum. A typical interchange follows.

Patient: "I thought if I waited long enough, my figure would be in fashion again. But I guess the days of Rubens and his corpulent ladies are gone forever."

Dr. Smith: "Culturally determined obesity does still exist. We could send you to Japan to become a sumo wrestler. Your special diet would allow you twice as much food as the Japanese average—exceeding 5,000 calories."

Patient: "I think I'd rather go back in time to the Kingdom of Kargwe in Africa where I would be forced to eat at the threat of being whipped, where 'fattening' was the first duty of a fashionable female life. But here we are in America in the late twentieth century. So what can you do for me, doc?"

Dr. Smith: "We can give you guidance. We can teach you how to approach the problem from a holistic perspective. But you have to do it for yourself.

"First, we need a clinical evaluation, perhaps a few standard test procedures, possibly a program of □stress□ reduction, and very definitely nutrition education."

Patient: "I'm sure you'll find out that my thyroid is perfectly normal, but that I suffer from overactive fork."

Dr. Smith: "That's an honest observation. Most patients tell me they eat far less than they actually do. That's one reason we don't take diets at face value, but search for hidden culprits."

Patient: "Don't some people gain inordinate amounts of weight disproportionate to what they are eating?"

Dr. Smith: "Oh, yes. There are many reasons for this. Among them:

1. Heavier people often gain more than thinner people on the same calorie content.
2. Metabolism slows as we get older.
3. Fine mechanisms of weight control may be disrupted after pregnancy.
4. The common □stresses□ of life may accelerate the deterioration of the relationship between thyroid and adrenal glands, which provide weight controlling feedback systems.
5. □**Drugs**□ (including □**nicotine**□) may stimulate metabolism; other □**drugs**□ (some tranquilizers) depress it.
6. Calorie intake may be identical, but the source may modify metabolism: has the food come from carbohydrates? From fats? Proteins? Are there a lot of □**processed**□ foods in the diet?

"Despite similarity of body type and body build, there could be a huge variation in intake."

Patient: "A few of the popular diets worked for me. Others didn't. A hundred pounds ago, I tried the thousand-calorie diet, but by 8:00 A.M. I had used up my calories, and it's a long day. I tried the Atkins diet. Instead of the ketone stick turning purple, my shoe turned yellow—I missed the stick. On the Stillman diet I got tired of carrying a bucket around. As for the Scarsdale diet, no wonder that lady shot that man.[2] Kidding aside, I usually lose when I start these diets, and then that's it."

Dr. Smith: "On a fad diet, you very often reach a plateau. This is due to an internal mechanism of thyroid function. The thyroid receives blood from your gut, which has absorbed your skimpy diet meal. The thyroid decides to hold back the burning of fuel because the fuel is so scarce on the 'starvation' regimen. It isn't the quantity that's missed, so much as the ☆**nutrients**☆. If the diet is undersized, but contains a bounty of nutrients, it responds differently. On inadequate nutrient intake, your thyroid slows the metabolism. It does this to conserve nutrients and maintain weight. The continuing starvation diet stresses the thyroid until it becomes exhausted. When this happens, you experience a sudden weight loss. You are thrilled to see the lower reading on the scale, but your joy is at the expense of the thyroid, a most important gland. One of its functions is the control of weight through hormone regulation."

Patient: "So what you are saying is that there is a control system dictating how much fat I should carry, and that fad diets disrupt this mechanism?"

Dr. Smith: "Everyone has an ideal body weight which is a *set point.* Although the quantity and quality of food you consume may have to do with many factors in your environment, your weight set point is controlled by genetic heritage, as are other set points like blood pressure, temperature, glucose level, pulse rate, respiration, sodium balances, and so on."

Patient: "Oh, so it's my thermostat ordering all that Chinese food?"

Dr. Smith: "Yes and no. There is a level of fatness, a physical structure, that your body strives to maintain. Your body, more than your mind, determines how fat you will be—all other things being equal. Your set point zeros in on the weight you would maintain (within a few pounds either way) if you were not dieting, or not cheating excessively.

"But there is also a familial predisposition to obesity which is more likely to relate to energy intake than to energy expediture.[3] This is in line with the observation that in many species food intake is determined by maternal example.[4] And obese dog owners tend to have obese dogs."[5]

Patient: "It sounds somewhat contradictory. A set point on the one hand, and learned habits on the other."

Dr. Smith: "Both of these factors are significant. You can maintain a relatively stable body weight even while the availability or caloric density of your diet is varied over a wide range. However, if given a rich and highly palatable diet, you may ingest many more calories and grow considerably heavier than you would if you were on a standard diet.[6] Overweight is a product of both nature and nurture.

"The activation of feeding behavior is determined not only by the stimulus of hunger, but also by gustatory and olfactory stimuli associated with food.[7] The accumulation of body fat can be either the result of increased food intake or the cause of it."

Patient: "Can I resist my set point in any way?"

Dr. Smith: "Not really. It's difficult to break the set point code. A Syrian woman has a different body structure than a Nordic woman. Instead of working within the idealized image of the thin, tall, emaciated fashion model, you need to work within the reference of your own set point. The body strives to return to this genetic marker. During illness, for example, the set point becomes unbalanced. The body depletes its fat reservoir, but it fights to come back to normal.

"No one can really say scientifically exactly what that set point is, but we do know that if you follow a judicious diet and live a life of equilibrium, your body will tend to go back to its original genetically prescribed weight, which may be more than you think it should be."

Patient: "Now he tells me. Where does that leave me and all the other poor overweight Americans?"

Dr. Smith: "Instead of resisting the set point, which can be such a potent and persevering competitive adversary, you can change it. For example, you can alter it unfavorably with □drugs□ or □sugar□, or you can modify it to your advantage with . . ."

Patient: "☆**Exercise**☆?"

Dr. Smith: "That's part of it. The total alternative, as presented in our modern concept of holistic health, is to study your body's constitution, explore your early and current life-styles, learn about previous illnesses and dysfunctions—everything that could be affecting your thermostat. And then we encourage you to get in the best condition possible, mentally and physically, and, yes, that includes ☆**exercise**☆."

Patient: "Can exercise alone lower the set point?"

Dr. Smith: "Yes. Your body composition changes when you exercise. Fat diminishes and lean muscle tissue increases. Muscle consumes considerably more calories to maintain itself than fat. Even if no weight is lost, a well-muscled person can ingest many more calories without gaining than a person who weighs the same but has less muscle tissue and more fat. It is speculated that exercise lowers the set point by raising the metabolic rate, and by altering body chemistry so that less fat is put in storage."[8]

Patient: "You said something earlier about honing in on personal dysfunctions. Would allergies interfere with my set point?"

Dr. Smith: "Yes. Most people crave those foods which are needed the least in terms of balance, in terms of the body's ☆**homeostasis**☆. Actually, there is no difference beween this and addiction. In fact, the food you crave has been called 'addictive' food, just like a □drug□. If we can cease thinking about food as food, and think instead about substances we are swallowing, we can better understand the mechanism of craving. It is not a physical need, but an actual desire. Compare, for instance, cravings for □heroin□, □coffee□, or □sugar□. These are addictive substances, all on the same level."

Patient: "I'm not sure I understand."

Dr. Smith: "Let me elaborate. It is undisputed that heroin is not a natural ingredient of the daily diet. You become conditioned to the 'high' of this physiologically addictive substance. After awhile, a vicious cycle has been set: in order to feel better, you have to keep introducing into your body that substance which will be harmful. The culprit is the very one used to ease the terrible symptoms. Everyone recognizes that this is heroin addiction. You respond in a similar fashion to ▫coffee▫ and ▫cigarettes▫. If you abstain from these abruptly, you have withdrawal symptoms. Perhaps a headache. Possibly extreme fatigue. When you have withdrawal symptoms, you feel better if you consume the coffee or smoke that cigarette, which compensates for the symptoms. And so it is with ▫alcohol▫. And so it is with ▫sugar▫. The symptoms of withdrawal can be worse than the symptoms caused by the intake of the addicting ingredient.

"Refined sugar is a man-made substance introduced as a food since childhood. Many people no longer have enough internal equilibrium for the pancreas, liver, and other glands to orchestrate the metabolizing of refined sugar. Before you know it, conditioning takes place exactly as in the case of any addictive drug response."

Patient: "So what you're saying is that we crave the very substances that are doing us in. I'm sure I've been involved in this vicious cycle ad infinitum. But you cited agents which are not 'natural.' What about nourishing foods? I know I'm sensitive to wheat, for example."

Dr. Smith: "And so it is with many foods. Nutrition researchers have found that the addictive syndrome does indeed occur with everyday foods. One example is gluten contained in some grains. It could happen with starches. Even tomatoes. In fact, commonly used foods are often the most allergenic."

Patient: "Getting back to my original question: what does this have to do with weight loss?"

Dr. Smith: "Ah, many people who have allergies have difficulty controlling weight. They do not understand that the problem is one of biochemical internal disarray caused by the food allergy, which interferes with the natural set point."

Patient: "How do you find out which foods you are sensitive to— which foods are interfering with weight loss?"

Dr. Smith: "We conduct very meticulous clinical evaluations through studies of eating habits, through nutrition analysis, and through whatever necessary avenues reveal the problem. Blood workups tell us about hormonal imbalances. Fasting glucose levels, cholesterol, and triglyceride levels may all point to problem areas."

Patient: "Is extensive testing always necessary?"

Dr. Smith: "Not in most cases. Simple screening, hair analysis (with expertise in interpretation), and nutritional analysis often guide us. The greatest value of the tests is that they graphically demonstrate your need to change your ways. It's very effective to show you a chart based on your blood chemistry. A colleague of mine sings 'Getting to Know You' as he analyzes his patients' blood.

"Elimination of the offending food or foods is of utmost importance. Add □**stress**□ reduction and an ☆**exercise**☆ program, and almost everyone loses weight—permanently. Lifelong awareness develops."

Patient: "If you discover my food sensitivities, and I make major changes, lose weight, and so on, will I ever be able to go back to the foods I've had trouble with?"

Dr. Smith: "Possibly. After a year or so of abstinence from foods you are sensitive to, we do introduce the offenders in small quantities as long as the food/patient/sensitivity/ratio is not very high. Our primary goal is to transform fatigued, rundown, and/or overweight individuals into healthy, vibrant people. The weight loss happens incidentally. Forty years of our changing foodways, which started after World War II, have not been a plus for your health or weight silhouette. Through the methods I've described, we can undo the damage."

Patient: "You have convinced me that I will lose weight if I follow all these life-style shifts. But how difficult will it be for me to make the changes?"

Dr. Smith: "It won't be easy. It has been said that one would sooner give up one's spouse than one's diet. In fact, according to Masters and Johnson, people would sooner give up sex than their diet. Lots of people don't have sex, but 'nobody doesn't eat junk food.' Seriously, the change requires incentive, vigor, and skill."

Patient: "Like that famous quote, 'If it is to be, it is up to me.' "

Dr. Smith: "Well said. But I can tell you one thing: It is unlikely that you will lose weight and keep it off any other way, with the exception of a routine ☆**exercise**☆ program. To encourage you, let me emphasize that a few months of brisk exercise, such as aerobic walking, can reduce a large percentage of fat accumulation that builds up in most people throughout their lives."[9]

Patient: "So if I didn't want to get involved in clinical evaluations and all that sort of thing, I could just exercise and keep the weight off?"

Dr. Smith: "Possibly. There may be two obstacles. (1) Many people start exercise programs and don't follow through. When you have to answer to someone, you are more likely to continue. (2) When exercising, energy is expended. You must be certain you are eating nutrient-dense foods. A poorly nourished cardiac muscle has to work much harder than a well-nourished one.[10]

"Sometimes all you need is one friend as a partner. If you start your aerobic program slowly, and increase the percentage of ☆whole natural foods☆ in your diet, you can certainly do it on your own."[11]

And that's how it goes. Day after day. Patient after patient. The more Bob examines the weight-control paradigm, the more convinced he is that recent research which explores the set point is explaining the most valid dieter's enemy. Imagine not being happy with your height and attempting to diet to lose or gain a few inches. This is no less frustrating than trying to lose weight with an elevated set point. Skeletal structure, tissue density, cell number, and even the desire for certain foods may be cemented in genetic and biochemical makeup.

When was set point fixed? Initially, millions of years ago along with other parameters. When is set point altered? The environmental overlay occurs at the moment of conception (or even prior to that), during the time of infant feeding, and throughout the rest of one's life.

Many people continue to fight valiantly, joining the diet-of-the-week club, losing a little, and gaining it back. With each retreat, the battle intensifies as the body maintains its set point (or even raises it). Just as one becomes thirsty to preserve sodium balance when consuming too much salt, so the body struggles to keep weight under control. It may not be what you consciously desire. *It is what your body wants.* There are differences in the efficiency of food energy utilization at a cellular level. For the lucky ones there is an increase in metabolic rate with an increase in food intake.[12,13]

For thirty years, a person is trying to gain ten pounds (a few of us). For thirty years, a person is trying to lose ten pounds (most of us). Or maybe even twenty pounds. Or thirty. Or more. With millions of years of genetics and a very young diet history behind the dieters, we make an advance here and there, but failure is inevitable unless each one changes his or her set point.

BEN'S COMMON SENSE CORRELATIONS

Semistarvation Studies

Ben is a story collector and historian. He has often read about experiments and anecdotes of forced diets during war years, and wonders why only the researchers have harnessed this information. He noticed, for example, that whenever Ida and his daughters went on rigid diets, they became irritable. And, of course, they replaced their weight rather quickly, as soon as the diet was terminated. He related their moodiness and diet failures to reports of semistarvation experiments, which took place during World War II. In these studies, when the subjects began to lose fat, they also became apathetic and fidgety. But when the experiment was ended, they ate with gusto, and the scales zipped back to normal, the subjects regaining all their fat.[14] Was this any different from Ida's starving on scoops of cottage cheese for three days, and then eating everything in sight on the fourth day?

When Ben shared his views of correlations between these experiments and his family's experiences, the response was, "What does that have to do with us?" Ben wonders why people think their bodies are different because they live in a different era, or because they have no common social reference points with a particular culture or group.

War Years and Food Insights

One of Ben's anecdotes concerns food deprivation followed by food quantity in Czechoslovakia after war years. The wartime exhaustion caused by reduced food intake, mental ▫stress▫, and hard work was soon compensated for by an outbreak of ▫obesity▫. A weight reducing regimen with a relatively rich caloric intake (1,800 calories a day) and very moderate physical activity, instituted in all hospitals and baths, turned out to be ineffective.[15]

Another story is unique in the annals of medicine. It is the report of a scientific investigation by physicians condemned to die of the same disease they were studying—hunger and subsequent starvation. Incredible observations by the Jewish physicians in the Warsaw ghetto brought to light information which is still being sorted out and analyzed, almost half a century later. The Nazis had sealed off several hundred thousand people from the outside world, determined to slowly starve them to death. The physicians decided to undertake a careful medical study of the consequences of hunger and starvation. Ben often discussed with friends the courage and persistence of the scientists, their despair, and the tragedy. The sophistication of these physicians is mind boggling. In the 1940s, they were recording observations that are currently being cited as new information. The studies were hidden and eventually smuggled out of the country.

Again, Ben wonders why it is taking so long for the assimilation and application of this kind of enlightenment:

- Blood sugar levels in hungry people are very low. Symptoms of hypoglycemia appear which are in accord with the modern concept that hypoglycemia stimulates sensations of hunger. (More than forty years ago these doctors understood the mechanisms of hypoglycemia.)
- Symptoms of hunger disease in test animals can be duplicated by feeding them a protein deficient diet.
- In hunger disease, the weight of the brain is unchanged, whereas heart, liver, kidney, and spleen are considerably lighter. (These doctors gave us important documentation of nature's protective priority for the brain.)
- Anemia, a condition so prevalent in our food-affluent country, was found only rarely in the Warsaw ghetto.
- Signs of vitamin deficiencies, which are characteristic in people on diets deficient in quality, do not necessarily occur in people whose diets are deficient in quantity. (This concept is almost entirely overlooked by today's establishment physician.)
- All of the young adults demonstrated early clouding of the lenses of the eyes similar to changes observed in senile cataracts. The assumption is that deficient nutrition is a very important factor in early lens clouding.
- When the diet consisted of black bread, oats, and kasha (buckwheat), there was very little vitamin B_1 deficiency, pellagra. This was not surprising because the ghetto diet contained ☆vitamin B☆.
- When confronted with hunger, the body manages its energy balance differently. The physiological demands of the hungry organism are somehow similar to those of animals hibernating in winter, when only a minimum of energy is used for work and moving around. Otherwise, their energy, which comes from burning their own tissues, would not last long. (This concept is helpful in understanding why fad diets don't work.)

- The metabolism of obese individuals differs markedly from that of lean or undernourished people. Since there is an abundance of adipose tissue in ◻**obesity**◻, the body is never required to utilize alternative energy sources.
- Cases of spontaneous recovery from diabetes were reported. There was also spontaneous recovery from various allergies and bronchial asthma. There was a marked decrease in the incidence of ulcers, gastritis, ileitis, liver and gall bladder disease. (When food is scarce, the first items to disappear are the junk foods.)
- During World War I, rickets was rampant. In the Warsaw ghetto, the children were poorly clothed and spent considerable time outdoors (often foraging for food). This exposure to sunlight was protective against rickets.
- The low fat diet dropped linoleic acid content below 1 percent of calories. Skin manifestations were those of essential fatty acid deficiency. (Here is another exquisite example of the avant-garde knowledge of these doctors.)
- The first stage of weight loss, when adipose tissue starts to disappear and skinfolds become shallower, produces a younger look. It is reminiscent of people returning from reducing spas, appearing and feeling younger and better. Unfortunately, the following stages of weight loss result in accelerated wrinkling and dryness, with overall aging.
- During the days of defeat and collapse of the city (Warsaw), men became impotent and many women stopped menstruating. When the diet returns to normal, these symptoms disappear rapidly. In undernourished patients, they remain. Many girls started menstruating upon receiving ☆**vitamin A**☆, even if they had not done so for a long time, or even if they had never menstruated because puberty started during the war.[16]

These studies represent extremes. But they do offer lessons. When the women in Ben's family embarked on each new fad diet (which Ben knew from the start would end in failure), he spoke of many things: cataracts and malnutrition; the slightly protective quality of ☆**whole foods**☆ even in the light of starvation; differences in metabolism; the importance of getting outdoors; skin conditions and essential fatty acid deficiencies. "Oh, Pop," they would say, "you just don't understand."

Ben understands a great deal. He also understands what we *don't* understand: limitation of knowledge in the area of hunger and weight control. Food consumption usually delivers caloric nutrients in amounts that far exceed immediate requirements. Therefore, most of our ingested nutrients are not utilized directly, but are incorporated into stores that are drawn upon after absorption has taken place. It is then, when the flux of calories from the intestines to the liver has diminished and the measured recruitment of stored fuels begins, that hunger seems to appear.[17] No one has really ever been able to identify the precise signal for hunger. It still isn't clear what specific event provides the initial stimulus that leads to food ingestion, where this event occurs, or how it is communicated to the brain.

Ben's Memories

Ben has fond memories of evening snacks and family comments.

"Maybe *your* cells need nutrients. But I am experiencing cheese cake deficiency right now."

"Of course I have to eat at night. Otherwise, I won't have the strength to sleep."

"I'm so glad I got over my recent illness. It was called 'dieting.' "

"So tonight I won't win the Nobelly Prize."

"Remember the à la mode!"

MIKE'S MIDDLE

Emotions and the Scale

Mike discovered that buying an automobile is the beginning of a spare tire. The first time he noticed weight gain was several months after acquisition of his first car. It was also a time of □stress□ in his life—he changed jobs, broke up with a girlfriend, and moved.

Mike was surprised to learn of the association between emotions and □weight gain□.

Many experiments show that animals will overeat when they are stressed, especially if the food is familiar, attractive, and readily available. (Fast food or Chinese restaurant after a hard day of work, anyone?) Animals can easily be taught to feed when exposed to an unpleasant stimulus.[18]

Not only does stress trigger overeating, but dieting may cause stress. It has been known for years that dieting can induce depression, even in apparently healthy, emotionally sound individuals. A lot more than fat goes down the drain. Loss of hair, loss of libido, loss of interest in other people—these are a few symptoms.[19] Instead of cutting down on calories, Mike stepped up his exercise program and began to eliminate specific food products.

The Milk and Wheat Connection

The food depletions were a consequence of data he was collecting on milk and wheat sensitivity. Only recently his mother told him he had been allergic to cow's milk formula as an infant. He has now been given information about correlations between milk and/or wheat and □stress□ and □**weight gain**□.

It has been shown that anxiety-induced overeating reflects the body's attempt to overcome emotional discomfort by increasing the concentrations of euphoric brain opioids—substances manufactured in the brain that make us feel good. This is accomplished via increased ingestion of gluten and casein, found in wheat and milk, and in any products made with them. The casein and the gluten act in the brain as morphine-like components. With repeated ingestion, they may become an addiction, just as morphine becomes an addiction. Consuming these substances actually creates a □**drug**□-like euphoria. Failure to get the "fix" causes symptoms not unlike withdrawal agonies, which prompt the "victim" to seek food—especially foods with gluten and/or casein: milk and cookies for Mike.[20]

One might conclude that this is the best of all ways to humor the body and get your kicks. Who would fault a milk-and-cookies junkie? Aside from throwing the set point askew (thus creating weight problems), there are other clinical manifestations from consuming foods to which you are sensitive. Among possible consequences are bloating, flatulence, irritable bowel syndrome, malabsorption difficulties (resulting from damage to the small intestine),[21,22] late menarche and earlier menopause in females, and higher incidence of infertility.[23] But there are very few disease states that are so easy to keep in check. A gluten- and milk-free diet is the antidote. It works like magic every time!

Fasting

A friend of Mike's encouraged him to fast. His friend said, "One day I put on my old army uniform, and the only thing that fit was the tie. I got involved in fasting, and I've never had another problem." Mike's friend explained that fasting creates a loss of appetite and an incredible feeling of well-being. Mike was hesitant. His friend continued to proselytize. He gave Mike several papers to read. One, by Judith H. Dobrzynski, stated:

Fasting has been around for centuries, since prehistoric times. Archaeologists have found ancient tablets mentioning it. The Bible talks about fasting on about seventy-five occasions. Socrates and Plato and Pythagoras did it to prepare for tests of their intellectual powers. Shakespeare weaves fasting into the blank verse of *Hamlet*, *The Merchant of Venice*, and at least three other plays. Franz Kafka wrote a short story about it, published in 1924.[24]

William Dufty, renowned journalist and playwright, relates the anecdote of a ship carrying a cargo of sugar. The vessel was shipwrecked in 1793. Five surviving sailors were rescued after being marooned for nine days. They were in a wasted condition due to starvation, having subsisted by eating nothing but sugar and drinking rum. Anyone who fasts will tell you that it is perfectly possible to survive safely for nine days or longer without food or water.

This incident inspired an eminent French physiologist to conduct a series of experiments with animals which he published in 1816. He fed dogs a diet of sugar or olive oil and water. All the dogs wasted and died, proving that some diets are worse than nothing.[25]

Mike questioned the health consequences of fasting. Fasting enthusiasts claim that since a faster resumes eating before too much lean tissue is lost, there's no harm done. Besides, when you are devouring your own body, your nourishment couldn't be better! Some doctors disagree, stating emphatically that fasting *must* be done under doctor's strict supervision. These caveats are issued:

- Many people may experience headaches, nervousness, faintness, or dizziness (especially when rising from a lying or sitting position).
- People with these conditions should not fast: heart disease, gouty arthritis, uncontrolled diabetes, anemia, and renal, cerebral, or hepatic disorders, or psychosis in remission. The same applies to anyone who is pregnant or is experiencing infections of any kind. (Is there anyone left?)
- The fasting patient has lower physical endurance.
- A good portion of the weight lost may come from the body's pro-

tein or muscle mass rather than from the body's excess fat reserves.[26]

- Reports of dangers, such as automobile accidents because of reduced acuity, have been noted.[27]
- Reports of physical problems abound. Gout or renal stones may be precipitated if fluid intake is insufficient; calcium and magnesium are lost; insulin decreases; hair growth may be arrested; and dry, scaly skin may develop. Fatty infiltration of the liver may occur.[28]
- Fasting exaggerates zinc deficiencies.

Fasting under the watchful eye of the physician is another story. Monitoring liquid intake, fasting with vegetable juices, partial fasts—these mitigate the problems. Dr. Allan Cott, renowned psychiatrist practicing orthomolecular therapy, who has fasted patients under hospital supervision, says:

It is a mistake to regard fasting as the panacea for whatever ails you. It is even a mistake to think of it as a cure for *anything*. But there is impressive documentation . . . that fasting allows the body to mobilize its defense mechanisms against many ills.[29]

Mike evaluated the pros and cons of fasting, and decided to shelve the idea for the time being.

Mike wasn't much impressed with protein sparing modified fasts, either. These diets may include solid protein in the form of lean meat, fish, or poultry. Liquid protein and powdered protein products are also available. Mike had read that even under medical supervision, adverse effects such as heartbeat irregularities could result from these diets.[30] Depletion of protein is a complex problem. Metabolic side effects of protein sparing fasts could be: diarrhea (initially), fatigue, cold intolerance, skin dryness, hair loss and muscle cramps.[31]

Mike is smart enough to know that most people revert to former eating habits following their protein product fasts. (Less than 10 percent weigh less than they did originally when checked after a few years.[32])

Richard Smith, who is so adept at poking fun, writes this about liquid protein diets:

"After three weeks on liquid protein, my husband didn't recognize me. After six weeks, I didn't recognize my husband."[33]

Mike's "tire" disappeared. He began to feel better and better. As he ran the track each day, he noticed that most "fatties" came and went. The "steadies" were lean and trim. Like Lovely Lady. Should he invite her to that new health food restaurant, or someplace more romantic?

MEG AND METABOLISM

The Scale and the Athlete

Meg is particularly interested in how exercise participates in weight loss and better body proportions. The numbers on the scale do not indicate how much of you is muscle or how much of you is *fat*. Meg has learned:

- In the absence of exercise, eating less does not prevent the occurrence of □obesity□. The opposite is also true. Exercise alone will not always decrease body fatness unless it is accompanied by dietary changes.[34]
- Increased ☆**physical activity**☆ in heavy work causes a proportional increase in food intake as compared to light work, but does not bring about any increase in body weight. On the other hand, when sedentary workers maintain the same caloric intake as heavy workers, their body weight is higher.[35]
- Excess calorie intake during early childhood can predispose a person to the development of excess fat. These adipose tissue accumulations could handicap the capacity for aerobic exercise.[36]
- Exercise plays an important role in fat metabolism and the regulation of body composition. For example, exercised animals deposit fewer fatty acids into fat tissue, even when measured twenty-four hours after the last exercise session. Reduced caloric intake does not compensate for a lack of physical ☆activity☆.[37] Deposits of fat in gymnasts *decrease* in spite of increased caloric intake when training is intensive, but *increase* after interruption of training, even when caloric intake is markedly reduced. Increased intensity of exercise causes the reduction of fat deposits in spite of the same relative weight of compared trained and untrained subjects. This applies to all age categories, from preschoolers to those of advanced age.[38]
- People engaged in static sports activities such as weight lifting and wrestling have such high fat ratios they could be classified as borderline □obese□. The highest level of weight and fat ratios is found

in sumo wrestlers. These athletes are often found to have elevated insulin and prediabetic tendencies. Fortunately, these values decrease with weight loss. Only specific kinds of exercise, however, can help reduce the fat ratio and the symptoms. (Another score for fast walking!) [39]

• In contrast to the athlete, a sedentary individual curtails the delivery of fat to skeletal and cardiac muscle, and boosts delivery to adipose tissue. [40] So if you're not moving around, your fat intake is added to your body fat, instead of going to places where it would be better utilized.

All this focus on adipose tissue stems from the fact that this is the site of energy storage. We know that when food is eaten in excess of energy requirements, storage occurs. Lack of activity slows the outflow of fat from adipose cells. Studies have shown a positive correlation between the blood flow per fat cell and the size of fat pads. Regular aerobic exercise reduces the size, but not the number, of fat cells.

Why do some people have more fat cells than others? Mother's diet during pregnancy may be a contributing factor. Any period of growth may lead to fat cell hyperplasia (increase in the number of cells). It is known that breast-fed babies weigh less and are shorter in length than bottle-fed babies. Forced feeding of infants may cause an overproduction of fat cells. The diet during weaning is especially significant. So, along with other things you blame on your mother, if you have too many fat cells, lay that on Mom too, especially since an increased number of these cells makes dieting difficult. [41] Muscle, by the way, leads to an increase in breadth of the chest and the proximal parts of the limbs (the parts situated nearest the point of attachment), while fat tends to increase abdominal dimensions.

The Mighty Mitochondria

Another positive benefit of exercise as it pertains to the diet/health paradigm started several hundred million years ago, when mitochondria were single-cell organisms living all by themselves. Mitochondria today are small components called organelles, which are found inside of cells. They are the principal sites of energy generation, resulting from oxidation of the food you eat. Your intake of sugar and fat and amino acids is broken down in these cells within cells.

The mitochondria are like the lungs of your cells—they transport oxygen and get rid of waste products. Now here's the interesting part: they have their own genetic continuity, containing an extranuclear source of DNA. They can divide without the parent cell dividing. The number of mitochondria can double or even triple under stress, and exercise is their best stressor. To function under the stress of exercise, or to meet the need of more oxidative machinery, the mitochondria increase in number. It's like having two or three times the lung power in your cells, allowing you to convert energy with more efficiency. When energy is more easily produced, fat is less likely to accumulate.

For mitochondria to be actively involved in energy production, high levels of ☆**B complex**☆ and ☆**trace elements**☆ are required. As energy production goes up, aerobic efficiency increases.[42] (This dispels a recent old wives' tale about B complex resulting in weight gain.)

If Meg's Mom is responsible for increased fat cells, she is also accountable for encouraging and supporting dancing lessons. And if Meg does have an overabundance of fat cells, you could have fooled Mike.

The two young men at the track were beginning to take on personalities. One is quite handsome, but, if a book is judged by its cover, a bit arrogant. The other has a pleasant, but not handsome face, a sunny smile and twinkly eyes. Meg likes twinkly eyes.

SALLY'S STRUGGLE

Carbohydrate Craving

The greater our advancement in technology, the smaller the bits and pieces available for examination. Sally's great-grandma associated fat people with "fat" foods. She used to say, "Broad noodles don't make narrow behinds." And that was that. (Except for Uncle Harry. He could eat a horse for lunch every day and not gain an ounce.) What would great-grandma say if she were told that brain mechanisms regulating protein and carbohydrate appetites involve serotonin-releasing neurons, among others? She would require a lot of 1980s science savvy before that would make any sense.

Simply (if that's possible), administration of a small carbohydrate-rich premeal causes an adjustment in food choices which increases the proportion of protein to carbohydrate selected in the total meal. Conversely, consumption of carbohydrate-poor, protein-rich meals—like those widely used for weight reduction—diminishes brain serotonin synthesis, thus increasing the desire for carbohydrate, often to the point of carbohydrate craving.[43] This may be another reason why Sally's dieting never worked.

Whether Sally views overweight as a complex process, the understanding of which requires the erudite backgrounds of M.I.T. scientists (thereby exonerating her from personal responsibility), or in the simple terms of great-grandma, Sally is just as unhappy saddled with excess weight. She has just begun to appreciate Victor Hugo's words, "Forty is the old age of youth; fifty the youth of old age." She wants to project a better image in her second youth.

When Are You Overweight?

What is overweight, anyway? Tables and guides are meaningless, because "average" weight may not be "normal" weight, nor may it be ideal weight, nor optimum weight. Dr. Reubin Andrés, clinical director of the Gerontology Research Center of the National Institute on Aging, concludes that a person is likely to be healthier weighing slightly above average. Dr. Robert J. Garrison, chief of biometric research at the Heart, Lung and Blood Institute, disagrees. A fascinating study explains why they are both right. Two groups of primitive people living near each other in South America were compared. The women in each group were overweight. One group enjoyed excellent health, despite obesity; the other was subject to all the degenerative diseases we know so well. Upon research, it was learned that the healthier group consumed a variety of whole foods. These foods were fattening, but natural. The ailing people were on a limited, more ▢processed▢ food plan. (Will we ever learn?)

Overweight patients usually know more about dieting than their doctors—unless the doctor happened to go on a few diets. Sally is aware that heavier people are "habit" eaters, consuming all that is readily available. Lean people, on the other hand, are readily influenced by their level of satiety and by past and anticipated activity. Gorging leads to greater hunger than does steady nibbling. Men allow substantial degrees of personal ▢obesity▢ to pass unnoticed, but women generally have a correct perception of their ideal body mass.[44,45,46]

Heat loss from the body of an overweight person is reduced by the thick layer of subcutaneous fat, which acts as an insulator. Since heat is kept in, calories are retained. Therefore daily energy needs are less than those of a slimmer person. But when a heavy person exercises, more energy is expended because there is a greater mass to move around.

Sally has learned that after slimming there is a lower energy requirement, which increases the likelihood of weight gain and explains in part the poor long-term results of many weight loss programs. To reestablish energy balance at a normal body weight, physical activity has to be increased to match the decreased metabolic rate.[47] That is why Sally is out walking the track each day.

With the exception of the exercising advantage, it appears that the odds are against anyone already overweight. As Sally says, "I don't gain weight between Christmas and New Year's, but between New Year's and Christmas. The other day I found myself asking a salesgirl if she had a larger dress in the same size."

Dangers of Losing and of Remaining Status Quo

Sally is well schooled in the liabilities of both losing weight and being overweight. She has learned that weight loss is associated with a marked loss of ☆zinc☆. If the weight loss diet itself has a low ☆zinc☆ content, this could be harmful. Many diet regimens encourage consumption of chicken, ☆fish☆, and ☆eggs☆ in place of red meat. But the zinc content of these protein foods is not adequate, especially since there are further zinc losses as weight is shed.

There are even differences in zinc content between different sections of chicken: the zinc content of light meat chicken breast is distinctly lower than the zinc content of dark meat chicken thigh. The quality of the meat also plays a role in providing zinc. The higher the fat content of the meat, the less zinc it contains.[48] Sally has acquired zinc know-how in her ongoing quest for the magic bullet reducing formula, although it is really of no great concern. She never stays on a diet long enough, and is very fond of nuts and seeds, which have plenty of zinc.

As for the inherent deleterious consequences of □overweight□ itself, Sally counts the ways:

- Women who are above 30 percent of ideal weight have a heightened sensitivity to pain.[49]
- The obese person never gets out from under the excess load. Even when sleeping, the excess weight on the abdomen pushes upwards on the diaphragm and compresses the heart and lungs.[50]

- Overweight people get two to four times the amount of heart disease, high blood pressure, strokes, cancer, and diabetes.[51,52,53]
- Overweight people have increased risks in many surgical procedures.
- The physical immobilization that accompanies arthritis is compounded in overweight people.
- Because the abdominal muscles are rendered less effective by the presence of fat, abdominal hernias are more common in the obese.[54]
- Anatomists say that we are still not adequately adapted to the erect posture (even when lean), and carrying extra loads is mechanically undesirable. Consequences include degenerative arthritis, particularly of hips, knees, and lumbar spine.[55]
- Obesity has long been recognized as promoting the development of cholesterol gallstones.[56]

It must be stressed that association is not proof of cause and effect. The quality of the food that adds pounds is paramount. (Rubens's ladies didn't get fat on candy bars and high technology pizza.) Obesity for many people may be irreversible, but positive dietary and life-style change advice is of great value. To tell an overweight person to avoid eggs and potatoes and to sprinkle bran on top of sugared packaged cereal will do nothing to help prevent the advance of the conditions listed. Nor will it do anything to reduce the pounds.[57]

In general, there is a low prevalence of diseases of civilization among populations where few individuals consume more than 2,500 calories per day. Adaptations to low intakes are known to increase longevity; adaptations to high intakes may carry a penalty.

Sally's closest friend has an incentive that works magnificently. Each time one of her children gets married, she slims down for the special occasion. Her friend bemoans the fact that she doesn't have a dozen children. As for Sally, she has her own bag of tricks, but they are not for losing. Among them:

1. Hide chocolate (well wrapped in foil) under the ice cubes. No one will ever think of looking there.
2. Eat in the bathroom. With the door locked, how could you ever be caught?
3. If you want a piece of cake, buy a small whole one, and eat all of it. That way, there is no incriminating evidence left. (Be sure not to leave crumbs.)
4. If you are ever caught in a compromising position with a bowl of

ice cream, say you blacked out—you just didn't realize what you were doing.

5. If you pull up to a fast food place for a quick snack, ask your spouse to stay in the car, and you run in for the food. Buy three frankfurters, and eat one before exiting the restaurant. Same maneuver works for doughnuts.

6. If the family orders take-out Chinese food, volunteer to pick it up. Upon arriving home, express shock at the inefficiency of the restaurant for giving you a container of chewed up spare rib bones.

7. Bake cookies for the neighborhood children. Of course you eat half of them yourself.

8. It is essential to have a dog. Then you can say, "The dog ate it."

9. After the party, say "You go to sleep. I'll clean up."

10. Double-wrap leftovers in heavy foil before discarding in case you want to retrieve them from garbage.

11. Buy cookies instead of cake. No one counts cookies, but missing cake wedges are apparent.

12. Be very charitable when it's Girl Scout cookie time.

13. If you polish off the remains of the peanut butter, open another jar and eat down to the level of the first jar, so no one will notice.

14. Swallow vitamin B_6 tablets two or three days in advance of a party to eliminate water retention. (You may lose a few pounds temporarily.)

While Sally is in the process of pulling it all together to look and feel better for the rest of her life, Shakespeare's lines from *Julius Caesar* are comforting: "Let me have men about me that are fat."

JANE AND JIM AND STAYING IN SHAPE

The Scale and the ▫Cigarette▫

▫Cigarette smoking▫ and ▫excess body weight▫, each of which contributes to poor health, appear themselves to be inversely related. Smokers generally weigh less than nonsmokers, and everyone knows weight gain occurs after cessation of smoking. The prospect of weight gain was a deterrent for Jim when he considered giving up his cigarettes, until: (1) The evidence against smoking was so strong, he could no longer ignore it. (Someone said, "If you continue smoking, Jim, don't buy any long-playing records or get involved in soap operas. You won't get to the end of either.") (2) Research indicates that smokers are not necessarily thin because they are eating less.

Some studies show that smokers may, in fact, consume more calories per day than nonsmokers. Smokers may be motivated to eat more to compensate for higher rates of metabolism and the less efficient use of calories that are consumed. Weight gain after stopping smoking could result, therefore, even without an increase in calorie intake. Its cause could be the more efficient absorption and reduced rate of metabolism of calories that are ingested. The smoker creates a variety of physiological effects that play a role in the amount of calories consumed per se.[58]

Toward Vegetarianism

When Jim stopped ▯smoking▯, he and Jane began to examine foods and calories and fats. Their diet began to change at this time, becoming more vegetarian. They ate more ☆**fish**☆, and less red meat. They included ☆**root vegetables**☆. These few changes alone had to bring nutritional profits.

They were impressed by an interesting study comparing weight losses of two groups of students. One group was encouraged to eat high fiber bread, and this group lost more weight than the control group, which ate ordinary ▯denatured▯ bread. The high fiber bread may have curbed hunger pangs enabling the dieter to resist foods that would have caused excessive caloric intake.[59]

Commercial breads available to Jane and Jim were not the high quality, high fiber variety they were looking for. They found several mail order bakeries that solved the problem, bought Essene breads at the local natural food store, and, for the first time in their lives, baked bread.

They compared foods, learning that most people with weight problems err in increments of 500 calories or more, the under-100 calorie differences between foods being inconsequential.[60] For example, drinking semiskimmed or skimmed milk is no health or weight advantage. A glass of skimmed milk contains about 88 calories and whole milk about 158.[61] Even if you drink several glasses a day, the total calorie saving is still under the significant five hundred. Don't you know overweight people who drink low-fat milk? And how long have they been drinking it? And how long have they been overweight?

Since the 70-calorie difference is not major, why consume a food in a more □processed□ form? This kind of milk product is highly unbalanced. Among other problems, fat is necessary for the assimilation of ☆calcium☆, and fat is sadly missing or in short supply in no- or low-fat milk. It has been shown that low-fat milk is harder to digest than whole milk.[62]

Despite so much evidence against low-fat milk products, millions continue to drink it, thinking they are consuming an especially healthful product. To paraphrase Anatole France, if fifty million people do a foolish thing, it is still a foolish thing.

Water Retention and The Scale

Jane had always suffered from water retention. Even when she ate very little, the scale could leap three to five, and sometimes even more, pounds the next morning. At a lecture given by Marshall Mandell, M.D., Jane heard the following:

You may not know if you are carrying a few or many pounds of excess water. The fluid retained in your body can be so evenly distributed, you may not be aware that you are waterlogged. Of course, if you have clearly visible puffiness of the eyes, face, or lips, or swelling of the hands, feet, or ankles, you will know.

These "bags under the eyes" are localized areas of "allergic edema." Allergic edema, or water retention, is one of the most misunderstood problems of overweight. It is a reversible disorder of the capillaries, those delicate, thin-walled blood vessels that carry nourishment to all parts of the body. During an allergic reaction, some of the fluid that is part of the blood plasma leaks through the allergically enlarged pores of the temporarily malfunctioning capillaries into the surrounding tissue, causing it to puff up with fluid. This is called "edema."

When the food or chemical that caused the allergic reaction is no longer present in the body, the walls of the capillaries return to normal and stop leaking fluid. The "allergic" fluid that has leaked into the tissues returns to the general circulation and is eliminated by the kidneys, excreted through the skin, or evaporated through the lungs, taking with it important pounds of unnecessary water weight in the form of allergic-edema fluid.

One type of edema that everybody has experienced is the mosquito bite. The female mosquito injects saliva in order to keep the blood from coagulating so that she can get a nice long free meal from the person she has bitten.

The body reacts to the mosquito's saliva by causing the capillary blood vessels at the site of the bite to dilate and leak a small amount of watery blood plasma into the surrounding tissues.[63]

Jane never did find out what foods caused her edema, but when she started her exercise program, eliminated "enemy foods," and made a few other changes in her diet, she no longer experienced water retention. More miraculously, her food cravings subsided. As explained earlier, allergy may be a pathway to obesity: if you eat foods you are sensitive to, it might ignite hunger.

A major problem is that any reminder of former substances of abuse produces instant cravings for the addict. Everyone is familiar with the conditioned reflex response demonstrated and popularized by Pavlov. It is no different when the sugar addict responds to the sweet taste of saccharin, which stimulates a fall in blood sugar. This is presumably caused by a conditioned reflex activation of the pancreas to secrete insulin. Avoiding the stimulus is virtually impossible. Sugar-containing foods are massively produced and promoted. It is difficult not to respond to all of the cues, especially when the main cue is *easy accessibility.*[64] (□**Artificial sweeteners**□ could drive up the set point, encouraging fatness. The sweeter they are, the greater the stimulation.[65] Beware of "new" sweetening agents.)

Food Encounters

Jane has been training herself to reencounter her "enemy foods" in various situations through a technique of directed imagination. For example, on signal, she imagines a dish of chocolate ice cream and immediately pictures the ice cream as glued into disgusting fat deposits in her stomach. The hope is that the vivid aversive response will block unwanted conditioned cravings. This "instant yuk" technique takes only a few seconds. She must also condition herself to see the successful outcome (not eating the chocolate ice cream) as a *gain,* not a *deprivation.*

Jane and Jim have pressed a few other "stock in trade" ideas into service:

- They became expert at preparing two gourmet dishes each. These meals are comprised of healthful ingredients only. The repertoire of four very special and delicious meals has made the transition easier. Each one is responsible for preparing dinner twice a week. The other meals are unplanned.

- Fat loss in a given energy expenditure is greater in a cold environment than in a warm one.[66] Reducing the house thermostat from 70 degrees to 68 is enough to make a difference.
- Liquids help fill you up. Jane and Jim drink plenty of water and include homemade soups in almost all meals.
- ☆**Nutrient density**☆ is more important than caloric density. Watermelon is more ☆**nutrient dense**☆ than a popular diet breakfast on the market.

  Lettuce contains almost all known nutrients. Although the nutrients are not in abundance, there is a wide range present, with protein representing 30 percent of the total in some varieties. Its value has been appreciated through the ages. Lettuce was served to ancient Persian kings, and it was popular with Romans. (Fresh-looking lettuce has more food value than limp, wilted leaves. Outer leaves contain more ☆**vitamin A**☆ and ☆**vitamin C**☆ than inner, lighter leaves.)

- Although Jane and Jim strive to serve fresh vegetables as frequently as possible, they always have bags of sautéed vegies in freezer packs, at the ready for soups, stews, and those "catch-as-catch-can" meals. Not as healthful as fresh, but a more healthful alternative to fast food places.
- While preparing breakfast, they cut up raw carrots, zucchini strips, cucumbers, green and red peppers, and so on, for nibbling—some to take with them, the remainder to eat when they return.
- They are rethinking their concepts of "fattening" and "nonfattening" foods. They had always thought of salmon and bananas as high-calorie foods. But most ☆**fish**☆ is extremely low in fat, and although salmon may have more fat than other varieties of fish, its fat content is no higher than that of many meats. Bananas do not contain any fat. Bananas have only 15 calories more than an equal amount of apple. The bland quality and soft texture of the banana, however, make it disappear so much faster.[67]

Dos and Don'ts That Don't Work

Jane and Jim are increasingly annoyed at the profusion of useless advice flooding magazines and books. Doesn't everyone know by now you might just as well spin wheels as:

Brush your teeth instead of snacking when you feel hungry
Keep your scale in the kitchen, instead of the bathroom

Set a timer for twenty minutes during mealtime (try this on a Type
    A personality who eats hurriedly and you'll have your head
    handed to you!)
Eat in front of a mirror
Keep a food diary
Eat only in one place
Never eat while on the phone
Look at yourself naked in a mirror each day
Avoid eating if you can't do it leisurely
Never eat dessert unless it's fresh fruit
Eat only with chopsticks
Wear tight clothing
Never eat in bed
Never eat standing up
Commune with each bite of food you chew

Why not speak to the wind, bay at the moon, or beat the air? At least these approaches will expend energy. The suggestions listed are made by doctors and reputable diet therapists every day. Is it possible they don't know these techniques won't work for more than 5 percent, if that many? (Or are they under contract to publishers, seeking "fluff" to fill their books?) There is such unprecedented attention to weight loss, and such precedented failure!

"'Tis not the meat, but 'tis the appetite
Makes eating a delight."[68]

KEITH AND CULTURE SHOCK

Then and Now

KEITH CUMMINGS I, 1925

Awakes to rooster and sun streaming in window. Goes to basement. Shovels coal in furnace. Boils water in kitchen for shaving lather. Sits at breakfast table. Shakes bottle of milk before pouring over hot cereal.

KEITH CUMMINGS III, 1985
(prior to running program)

Awakes to digital clock on ceiling. Uses electric razor, electric toothbrush, electric hair dryer, automatic water pic. Sits at breakfast table. Pours cereal from box, milk from container, coffee

Walks one mile to office. Walks, runs, stands all day on job. Walks to various stores to purchase supplies. Walks home. Sits down to dinner. Paints front fence. Repairs chair. Works on tree house with children. Walks six blocks to visit friend. Walks home. Knock on door informs of phone call. Walks to store, two blocks away, to receive call. Walks back. Goes down to basement. Shovels coal. Banks furnace for night. Dreams of sitting on deck of ocean liner for ten days.

from automatic percolator, which started before he awoke. Shines shoes with electric kit. Sits in car, headed for RR. Arrives early in order to park close to RR entrance. Sits on train. Sits in taxi. Takes elevator to office. Sits in large swivel chair. Swivels to reach files in rear. Secretary brings additional files; dials all phone calls. Computer terminal on desk facilitates procurement of data from other departments. Coffee served at desk, while on phone. Sits in taxi to RR station. Sits on train. Sits in car. Sits down to dinner. Sits in front of TV. Answers phone through TV. Sits in bathtub. Uses cordless phone to answer call while in bathtub. Gets into bed, adjusting mattress to upright position. Uses remote control for turning TV on and house lights off. Falls asleep. Dreams of coming in first in major marathon meet.

Keith has often wondered which overweight relative he takes after. It could not have been Grandpa Keith. Look at that picture of gramps at the same age. How slim and trim he was! Although Keith had never associated his personal scale readings with lack of body movement until his adventures on the track, he has conjectured about this age of high technology. What else could be automated? "Please," he says, "don't automate sex. I'd rather do that myself."

Loser's Library

Before Keith's jogging days, he attempted to keep in rank by using every scheme in every diet book. He started with a few journals found in the family library, discarding one set of cunning and crafty lose weight stratagems for the newest get-the-scale-down maneuver, hot off the press. No plan was so clever that he ever achieved his goal: the lean-as-a-rake-Grandpa-Keith look. Here are excerpts from his "Loser's Library":

Banting's Diet, William Banting, 1853:

"Of all the parasites that affect humanity, I do not know of, nor can I imagine, any more distressing than that of obesity, and having just emerged from a very long probation in this affliction, I am desirous of circulating my humble knowledge and experience for the benefit of my fellow man with the earnest hope that it may lead to the same comfort and happiness I now feel under the extraordinary change— which might almost be termed miraculous had it not been accomplished by the most simple common-sense means." (The Banting diet was basically high protein, a diet adopted by Stillman and Atkins. We're glad Stillman and Atkins didn't mimic Banting's penchant for long sentences.)

Tomorrow We Diet, Nina Wilcox Putnam, 1922:

The author blames the fact that she overstepped the line between "cuteness and corpulency" on the advent of the car.

1. Don't pull, "Well, I will take a little just this once."
2. When dieting in public, sneer at the waiter before he sneers at you.
3. White bread is low in nutrition. A federal experiment showed that birds fed on white bread and water dropped and died.
4. Have bran three times a day. It contributes to loss of flesh and to the general betterment of your entire physical condition. Have two bran crackers with each meal. That's an order.
5. We eat too much, too often, and too stupidly. Which do you chose: "I want to be slender," or "I want the custard pie."
6. Order steak, chops, roast veal, or broiled kidneys. Ask that your fish be broiled. Order lettuce, string beans, and fruit. It is fashionable to order a small coffee.
7. Do not have any alcohol, potatoes, nuts, sugar, bacon, milk, sauces, grapes, bread.
8. Buy a "shimmy" chair.
9. Take Slimlin's (the Physician's Pellette). Three a day take your flesh away.

(Note that the date of this book is 1922. Here we go again: nothing's new under the sun!)

The New Way to Eat and Get Slim, Donald G. Cooley, 1941:

1. ▫Coffee▫ and ▫tea▫ can never make you fat. Your reducing diet allows you to consume them until you splash when you walk. Have black coffee and clear tea.
2. To provide skim milk for your reducing diet, simply pour off the cream from the top of the milk bottle.

Diet Does It: You Are What You Eat, Gayelord Hauser, 1944:

1. You may never get the amount of ☆vitamin A☆ needed to build vital health and to give full zest for life.
2. Avoid: devitalized foods, soft drinks, pastries, jams, jellies, white flour, and refined sugar.
3. The vital diet: three glasses of ☆yogurt☆ daily, an ☆egg☆ or two, cottage cheese, ☆liver☆, heart or sweetbreads, kidneys, brain.
4. ☆A☆ and D capsule from fish-liver oil; ☆B☆ from ☆brewer's yeast☆, wheat germ, and black molasses. Brewer's yeast is acclaimed the greatest food discovery of all time.
5. Combine celery and carrot juice. We now know there is a nutrient factor in carrots that reduces the body's need for oxygen. There is an antifatigue nutrient in liver and wheat germ oil.

(Perhaps we should pay special attention to this section. Hauser is in his late eighties, and still going strong.)

Calories Don't Count, Herman Taller, M.D., 1961:

1. You have before you the solution to your weight problem. Now you must begin to do things for yourself.
2. The key substance in vegetable oils is linoleic acid, an essential fatty acid. The more oil you drink, the more body fat you will burn. Safflower oil is the most valuable.
3. The less carbohydrate you eat, the less body fat you will produce.
4. You do not have to count calories, but do not eat *any* of the foods that are not permitted.
5. Make sure that you eat fish or seafood once a day, because marine food is rich in unsaturated fatty acids.
6. Don't worry about taking in too much fat. Your body will let you

know when you have had enough. (The sign of eating too much fat is nausea.)

7. Avoid salt and alcohol.
8. Do not check your weight on a scale. We are treating obesity, not overweight. The fit of your clothing will tell you how successful you are.
9. Walk at least one hour every day.

(Taller was actually prosecuted for his ideas.)

The Expense Account Diet, Jonathan Dolger, 1969:

Check-Grabbing and Other Exercises

1. The greatest potential source of exercise in the Lunch Business is, of course, walking to lunch. Pick a restaurant at least five blocks away.
2. The other main source of exercise in the Lunch Business is signing the check. Depending on your style and instrument, check-grabbing can be a profitable way to take off a few extra pounds.
3. If you find yourself alone in the elevator going back to work, do the Charleston.

Did You Ever See A Fat Squirrel?, Ruth Adams, 1972:

1. Obese individuals may actually be malnourished.
2. Once an animal becomes obese, it becomes obese more easily and more rapidly a second time.
3. People whose weight has fluctuated up and down a number of times have been subjected to more atherogenic (condition in which fatty deposits form in the arteries) stress than people whose weights are stable.
4. While only 12 percent of all women in their twenties are dreadfully overweight, 45 percent of all women in their sixties are obese.

Dr. Atkins Diet Revolution, Robert Atkins, 1972:

1. You can eat as much as you want as long as it is high protein and fat, and low carbohydrate.
2. If you can't give up drinking, then you'd better admit you have a drinking problem. It is unlikely that your weight problem will be solved if your drinking problem is not.
3. Taking a diuretic seems to be a favorite way of cheating with over-

weight. Remember, it takes the water off, but leaves the fat behind.

4. The worst feature about this diet is the rapidity with which you
gain if you abandon it. But the best feature is that you don't have
to go off this diet.

The Beautiful People's Diet Book, Luciana Avedon and Jeanne Molli,
1973:

1. Maria Callas walked around with a calorie book.
2. Van Johnson put a picture of Audrey Hepburn on his refrigerator.
(You know, all hollows and bones.)
3. Cristina Ford has an Italian grocer come every day at 8:00 A.M.
with fruit and vegetables in season—at its freshest.

The Bronx Diet, Richard Smith, 1979:

1. The dedication page:
"O, that this too too solid flesh would melt . . ." (Act I, Scene
II, *Hamlet*)
"Bring on the eats!" (Act I, Scene I, Bar Mitzvah of Sid Boren-
stein)
2. A Twinkie contains twice the restfulness as that found in a pound
of calf's liver.

How to Stay Slim and Healthy on the Fast Food Diet, Judith Stern
and R.V. Denenberg, 1980:

1. The skin is the best part of Kentucky Fried Chicken, but you can
save about 100 calories just by peeling it off.
2. Strawberry ice cream has 141 calories per scoop compared to 181
for French vanilla. Skip the sugar cone. That has 40 calories.
3. While dieting, the only part of the donut that is safe to eat is the
hole. Dunkin' Donuts invented Munchkins, which are little round
pastries with no fillings. Almost half of its calories are from fat.

Short Rations: Confessions of a Cranky Calorie-Counter, Joan M.
Scobey, 1980:

1. There's nothing like trying on blue jeans to bring you back to reality. Just when you think you're so thin.
2. At my before-breakfast, no-clothes weigh-in, my scale is wavering

between 140 and 141. Add 2 pounds for the doctor's scale, and it doesn't bode well. I feel like I'm on my way to the principal's office.
3. There was Christmas Day, several New Year's celebrations, and even a bar mitzvah slipped in. Three pounds.

The Pritikin Permanent Weight-Loss Manual, Nathan Pritikin, 1981:

1. Snacking between meals is definitely approved on the Pritikin diet. At the Centers, food is offered at eight different times during the day. The body functions best when food is taken at closer rather than more spaced-out intervals.
2. Adherence to a high-protein diet usually results in initial weight loss, but the loss is not permanent. It is due primarily to large amounts of water lost from the tissues because the body is trying to eliminate the dangerous byproducts of the large amounts of protein ingested.
3. Much maligned carbohydrates turn out to be not only the healthiest kinds of foods we eat, but also the kinds that keep people slim.

F-Plan Diet, Audrey Eyton, 1982:

1. Never let anyone, or any diet, convince you that calories don't count in achieving weight loss. They do. They are what reducing is all about.
2. Sometimes just a few dashes of olive oil and a sprinkling of lemon juice, along with salt and herbs, will provide all the dressing you need.
3. Fruit juices are not allowed on the F-Plan. They are simply fruit stripped of its natural fiber content. When you drink orange juice you are getting all the calories that are present in the orange in the form of sugar, with none of the fiber-filling power.

It's Not Your Fault You're Fat Diet, Marshall Mandell and Fran Gare Mandell, 1982:

1. Meals, including snacks, must be at least four hours apart. With some food-allergic individuals, it takes a minimum of three to four hours for them to fully react to an allergic offender. You may not know which foods are bothering you if you don't allow this amount of time to elapse between feedings.

2. When you are going to be away from home, make sure you carry with you all of the foods you will need for the day, so you won't become too hungry and be tempted to go off your diet.

The Hamptons Health Spa Diet Cookbook, Florence Kulick and Florence Matthews, 1983:

1. When driving a car or sitting at a desk, contract your abdominal muscles to the count of five and then relax to the count of five. Repeat several times. This is good for tightening your stomach muscles.
2. Tighten your buttocks while preparing a meal, doing housework, or washing the car.

When Keith hooked into any one of these regimens, he was absolutely rigid, uncompromising, and strict, except when it was time for: coffee breaks, business meetings, two-martini lunches, weddings, dinner parties (his or friends'), holiday celebrations, dates, carnivals, picnics, vacations, business trips and/or conventions, dinner at his mom's, baseball games, TV football viewing on Sunday afternoons. And, oh yes, if he happened to pass a hot dog stand. . . . Keith, like many, "can resist everything except temptation."

His final failure was a short-lived relationship with a salon on Wall Street whose advertisements read, "REDUCING FOR STOCKY BROKERS."

But no matter. Now that Keith was exercising and thinking about decreasing ◻**nicotine**◻, all would be well with the world and his weight. He was slimming down (again). And wasn't that cute chick at the track giving him a message? Maybe The Four Seasons for dinner, and then a nightcap at Sardi's. . . .

> My candle burns at both ends;
> It will not last the night;
> But, ah, my foes, and, oh, my friends—
> It gives a lovely light.[69]

CHAPTER 4

Food Consequences

The new bride was preparing her first roast beef dinner. Before placing it in the oven, she sliced off the end. "Why'd you do that?" asked her husband. "Doesn't everyone?" she answered. "Mom always cuts the end off the roast." "That's silly," he said. "And expensive. Let's call Mom and find out why she does that." "Gee," said Mom when they called, "Grandma always eliminated the end of the roast beef. I thought everyone did." More confused than ever, the young man called Grandma. "Grandma, please explain why you cut the end off the roast beef." "Simple," answered Grandma. "I cut the end off because it doesn't fit in the pan."

BOB SMITH'S CONFERENCE: BEYOND MEDICINE

Even A Lemon Can Be A Lemon

Bob had a "vacation" feeling as he traveled at 30,000 feet on a 747. Destination: medical convention. After settling as comfortably as possible in his confined space, he pulled out a few medical journals saved for the occasion. Bob was especially impressed with an article called "Nutrition, Health and the Future," by Walter Yellowlees, a Scottish Highlander:

Aberfeldy is a place of unsurpassed beauty. Our valley of good farming lands runs east and west and is enclosed by steep-sided hills which rise to heather-covered moors and forest. The landscape is a superb harmony of fields, rivers, mountains, and lochs.

106

I tell you this not as a commercial for any who are planning their next summer holiday in Scotland, but because the quiet beauty of the place is of great importance when we ponder on the causes of the common disease daily encountered in general practice. Visitors, sometimes medically qualified visitors, are apt to explain as they gaze on the marvelous vista, "But surely there is no need for a doctor in a place like this?"

They echo the widely held belief that many modern diseases of our time are caused by the rush of urban living, by executive type □stress□. If urban stress were an important cause of diseases like duodenal ulcer, coronary thrombosis, or high blood pressure then their occurrence would be rare in Aberfeldy.

Alas, this is not so. These diseases are common in the modern Highlander. . . . Dental decay, diabetes, obesity, varicose veins, disordered bowel function, peptic ulcer, coronary heart disease, high blood pressure and, above all, cancer are encountered daily in the surgery.

. . . When visiting patients at mealtimes I have been repeatedly appalled at what I saw on the family table. Tinned meat, tinned vegetables, very seldom any salads, masses of white bread, scones, biscuits, cakes, sweet drinks, packeted milk puddings, margarine instead of butter, and seldom porridge now, mostly the ubiquitous packeted sweet breakfast food.[1]

> "O, that deceit should dwell
> In such a gorgeous palace"[2]

Bob felt a kinship with this doctor, another general practitioner who recognizes the unique opportunity of observing the daily lives of patients. Yellowlees concludes, "Until our people can enjoy food which is fresh, varied, unrefined, and grown on fertile soil, our health is not likely to improve."

The changing food consumption in the Scottish Highlands parallels that in any suburb or city of America. Bob recalled an experience he had exactly a year ago, attending the same convention. He took time out to photograph endless groves of sparkling oranges and lemons. After packing his camera, he entered a pretty little restaurant just off the Pacific Coast Highway. He could still sense the bright sun bouncing off the dazzling yellow fruit as he sat waiting for his lunch, and he thought of the advantages of living on the West Coast: surely *this* citrus fruit must have its full complement of ☆**vitamin C**☆. As he pondered whether or not he would need vitamin C in supplemental form if he lived in California, he playfully picked up a packet, one of many, which was sitting in a bowl on the table. The packet read: "For your reconstituted lemon." The packet contained *dried* lemon and a potpourri of additives—right smack in the middle of a great profusion of lustrous lemon trees!

In his article, Yellowlees quotes from *The Deserted Village*:

"A bold peasantry, their country's pride,
When once destroyed, can never be supplied."[3]

And from *The Rape of the Earth*:

"Men are permitted to dominate nature on precisely the same condition as trees and plants, namely that they improve the soil and leave it a little better for posterity than they found it."[4]

Vegetarian Vexations

The sound of his name separated Bob from the article. He had been so engrossed, he hardly heard the dinner trays snapping into place. "Passenger Smith?" He identified himself, and was handed a special meal.

Bob dubbed airplane food "reruns" because of their similarity to leftover TV dinners, and jokes about the possibility of breaking out in test patterns when subjected to too many of them. Despite the fact that you've paid for the meal, you can't even send it back or demand a refund when it's unsatisfactory. Finding airline food so distasteful, he often bags his own. But someone had given him a tip: Call twenty-four hours ahead and order a special dinner. It's usually better than the platter of the day.

Bob did just that, and selected "vegetarian" from among the choices. On this trip, the passengers were enjoying chicken, rice, and broccoli, with rolls and butter, all of which looked and smelled better than most meals he had seen 30,000 feet above ground. But today the saddle was on the wrong horse: Bob could not believe the offensive provisions set before him. Two slices of white bread, a cup of commercial peanut butter, a cup of jelly, a cup of margarine, several slices of processed cheese, nondairy cream for coffee, and a piece of cake with a label that stated: "No butter, milk, or cream in this product."

What a sad misinterpretation of vegetarian food. A well-planned vegetarian diet should be consistent with good nutritional status. At the very least, it should resemble something that once grew in the ground. A poor assortment of vegetarian food could increase the risk of diet-related disorders. The people putting these provisions together see vegetarianism as abstinence from animal foods. Period.

The popularity of vegetarian diets is greater today than at any time in our history. Apparently the forms that have emerged may differ strikingly from traditional vegetarian patterns. The vegetarian diet which includes unprocessed ☆vegetable☆ and other plant foods is being heralded in every medical journal:

Journal of the American Dietetic Association: Even though the concentration of essential amino acids in plants is lower, if the amino acids in ☆vegetable☆ mixtures are supplied in appropriate proportions, they are as effective at minimum levels in meeting the body's needs as proteins from animal sources.[5]

New England Journal of Medicine: Relatively high intakes of dietary fiber are characteristic of vegetarians. An increase in fiber content has been reported to have beneficial results.[6]

American Journal of Clinical Nutrition: Diabetes improves with high-fiber, ☆complex carbohydrate☆ diets, typical of vegetarianism.[7]

American Journal of Clinical Nutrition: Low folate blood levels are not uncommon, even in apparently healthy people. Folates are destroyed easily in cooking. Since folate is present in large amounts in ☆vegetables☆, vegetarians usually have normal or even high blood values of folate.[8]

Lancet: Chronic arthritis has been associated with low levels of pantothenic acid. Vegetarians have more pantothenic acid than those on average American diets.[9]

Lancet: There is a hypocholesterolemic effect of vegetable protein. Hypocholesterolemic means low cholesterol. When patients with high cholesterol levels consume ☆vegetable☆ foods, cholesterol drops.[10]

American Heart Journal: Patients with severe angina pectoris benefit from a vegetarian diet.[11]

Bob would like to recommend a pure vegetarian diet to many of his patients as a therapeutic regimen for serious problems. This excludes all animal foods in any form, and includes unusual and extraordinarily healthful vegetarian foods. But it takes a lot of life-style change to arrive at this kind of daily menu, an example of which is:

Breakfast: Buckwheat porridge with sesame seed milk, berries, and small quantity of soaked, dried fruit. Fresh fruit and lentils and flax seed, or their ☆**sprouts**☆.

Lunch: Raw foods: tomatoes, cucumbers, finely minced carrots, green and red peppers, green leafy ☆**vegetables**☆, fermented mixed ☆**vegetables**☆, cabbage; mixed salads of: steamed or raw beets, potatoes, parsley, garlic; ☆**cultured milk product**☆.

Dinner: Raw foods and mixed salads and a hot soup boiled from ☆**roots**☆ and ☆**vegetables**☆. Soup is served with bread (buckwheat rolls, crisp hard rye bread, or Essene, which is ☆**sprouted**☆ wheat or rye bread).

Snacks: Herb teas, fruit, and vegetable juices served at room temperature. Small quantity of nuts and seeds.

This is a rather stringent vegetarian dietary regimen. Needless to say, Bob was not expecting anything remotely resembling such a meal plan on the plane. But he did anticipate an ☆**enzyme**☆ or two. Instead, he was served highly □**processed**□, additive- and trans-fat laden nonfoods. (*Trans*-fats are explained later in this chapter.) He decided he could get more nourishment biting his lip.

Margarine Mayhem

Too many of Bob's patients are under the misconception that margarine is nutritionally superior to butter. For this reason, he prepared a fact sheet on the subject. Bob often uses fact sheets for patient education.

Since a caricature is a likeness or imitation that is so distorted or inferior as to seem ludicrous, Bob labeled this paper "The Butter Caricature: Margarine." Most of the information in "The Butter Caricature" comes from the writings of three people who have done an incredibly fine job of informing America about food deceptions. They are Beatrice Trum Hunter, Rudolph Ballentine, M.D., and Jeffrey Bland, Ph.D. The balance of the material has been gleaned from "establishment" medical journals. Dr. Smith's clinical experience confirms the views expounded.

THE BUTTER CARICATURE

When margarine first appeared on the market, sales were low. Margarine looked and tasted like lard. Back to the drawing board! Margarine was then sold with a coloring agent for esthetic improvement. But people didn't want to color their own food. Back to the drawing board! Sophisticated techniques emerged, and with them, margarine that looked, smelled, and tasted like butter. Believe it or not, now it was the butter industry that went back to the drawing board. Today most butter contains color □additives□ to compete with the "yellowness" of margarine.

Margarine is often advertised as being derived "from polyunsaturated oils." Manufacturers neglect to mention that the oil is changed into margarine by hydrogenation—saturating it with hydrogen. Some margarines do contain small amounts of liquid polyunsaturated oil added to a hydrogenated base, but the bulk of the fat must, of necessity, be saturated. Otherwise the margarine would be liquid like any other polyunsaturated oil.

Once a vegetable oil is hydrogenized, however, a new fat has been created. Such artificially hydrogenated vegetable fats are a recent addition to the diet. The human body has had no experience with them. It seems reasonable to wonder if we have the capacity to deal comfortably with this essentially synthetic food.

In fact, elaborate statistical analysis of the incidence of heart disease and the consumption of hydrogenated fats in England has shown a dramatic and detailed correlation between the two. Where margarine and solid vegetable shortenings are used in significant quantities, the rate of heart attack is always higher than where they are not.

Margarine is a perfect example of a fabricated food, the earliest nondairy substitute. Manufacturers invested large sums of money for research in the technique of "creaming" margarine to increase the public's acceptance of the product. A survey has shown that advertisements have influenced consumers' choices for margarine over butter.

The advertising campaign launched by margarine manufacturers was termed "one of the most unprincipled food promotions in the past quarter of a century," with TV commercials described as "noisy, ubiquitous, and shameless." They have promoted a staple food as though it were a drug. Margarine advertisements were directed especially to physicians. Physicians, lacking information about how the hydrogenation process affects human health, or about the hazards of too much □processed□ polyunsaturated fat, began switching patients from butter to margarine and from animal fats to vegetable oils.

Hydrogenated fats have a higher melting point than fats that are liquid at room temperature. They are less well utilized in your body. They do not circulate in the blood or move through the tissues as liquids. They may disrupt the permeability characteristics of the membranes of the body's cells and prevent the normal transport of nutrients into and out of cells.

Hydrogenated fats produce a deficiency of essential fatty acids (EFA) by destroying them, or producing abnormal toxic fatty acids. Deficiency of EFA is a contributory cause in neurological diseases, heart disease, arteriosclerosis, skin disease, various degenerative conditions such as cataract and arthritis, and cancer.

The conversion of oils to the hydrogenated form actually prevents the proper formation of bile in the liver from cholesterol, and therefore can elevate blood cholesterol and have adverse effects both directly and indirectly. *Margarine can raise cholesterol.*

The Butter Information Council, in a campaign to encourage people to eat more of their products, has introduced a booklet on butter, informing the public that:

1. Butter is a natural product—alternatives are different.
2. All butter is made with cream. The ingredients of margarine are varied in individual brands.
3. Butter is a healthful food. There is no evidence to the contrary.
4. Butter has been in the diet for thousands of years so you can have confidence in it.
5. Butter is no more fattening than margarine. This is an important point. The advertising of margarine has been so powerful and misleading that it is surprising how many people still think margarine has fewer calories than butter. Again, *the fat content of butter and margarine are identical.*
6. Fats are important in a well-balanced diet.[12,13,14]

A study reported in the prestigious journal *Atherosclerosis* reports that neither milk, cream, cheese, nor butter have any consistent effect upon blood cholesterol.[15] George V. Mann, one of the first to call attention to the misleading margarine propaganda, has shown that a change from butter to margarine may be harmful.[16] An article in *Lancet* reports that most popular brands of margarine are highly saturated and some contain more cholesterol than butter.[17]

In test studies with nonhuman primates fed peanut, coconut, butter, and corn oils supplemented with cholesterol, the most severe atherosclerotic lesions were produced by peanut oil and next came coconut oil, with butter trailing behind.[18]

Trans-fats are formed as a result of chemical hydrogenation. They are artificially created, and margarine may contain up to 45 percent of these deleterious fats. Only in recent years have *trans*-fats formed a significant part of our diet. Can a food containing this high level of *trans*-fats be more healthful than butter?[19]

A proliferation of articles express these scientific facts in recent issues of medical journals. But as Voltaire said, "It requires ages to destroy a popular opinion."

Butter (and eggs) are the innocent victims of the fervor of the evangelical zest of the anticholesterol establishment which attempts to replace proved foods with untried substitutes.[20]

—Bob Smith, M.D.

Homeward Bound and a Few Missed Concepts

On the return flight, it was difficult for Bob to concentrate on reading. He had learned so much, and been irritated by more. His medical colleagues appeared to have little interest in the subject of nutrition. Yellowlees had said, "The general practitioner who tries to wage war on this dreadful dietary regime finds the fight a lonely business . . . So our national disease service continues to be one of the few growth industries in the land."

At the banquet dinner, Bob mumbled something about the ersatz cream served with □coffee□. A colleague retorted, "Cream to the physician means concentrated saturated fat and cholesterol." This is not what it means to me, thought Bob. It means lots of ☆**vitamin A**☆, and phosphorus, ☆**calcium**☆, a dash of magnesium, and some riboflavin. And oh, yes—cream also means strawberries.

There was no use informing his dinner partner that the make-believe cream:

1. whitens better, so the customer doesn't use as much
2. stays perfectly fresh for three weeks under normal refrigeration
3. stays on the table up to three hours
4. includes an astonishing array of ingredients, mostly chemicals
5. may consist of sucrose (sugar) and corn syrup solids as sweetening agents
6. contains fat which is usually coconut or palm kernel oil, both of which are highly saturated, thereby totaling more saturated fat than is found in the butterfat of milk
7. may contain at least as many calories as whole milk[21]
8. in Bob's mind is more closely related to paint than food

Bob was sorry he commented at all. He has no personal interest in nondairy creamers. He doesn't even drink coffee.

Someone casually mentioned the scientific documentation of garlic and its beneficial effect on blood pressure. Bob shook his head in despair as he thought of the doctor's comment: "I'd much rather treat my high blood pressure patients with □**drugs**□. When I prescribe drugs, I can control the amount. Who knows how much garlic a person will take?"

"I can control." The doctor must be captain at all times. The drug is standard, but what about the patient? Weight variations? Metabolic differences? Diet and drug synergism? Perhaps the doctor thinks all meals should be encapsulated. Then the doctor could control it all!

Bob recognizes that the doctor is not entirely at fault. Bob, as a physician, is in one of the most privileged positions in the social order of the world. Doctors do save lives and help bring them into the world. They make life more (and sometimes less) comfortable, and may even, by error or ignorance, hasten the death of a patient. This is □**stress**□. Some physicians cope by adopting a controlling, directive stance with patients. The physician-God may hide from life behind a mask of unlimited authority and knowledge. And patients themselves project a superhuman power on the doctor. It is difficult for the doctor to avoid absorbing this attitude.[22]

At the prebanquet cocktail party, one of the doctors offered aspirin as though he were handing out Lifesavers. "Don't you know that aspirin and □**alcohol**□ may prevent heart disease?" His comment was given the stamp of implied credibility when he cited the source of this information, namely, the *New England Journal of Medicine*. Bob was familiar with the report, which described in sound fashion the ability of alcohol to augment aspirin-induced increases of bleeding time. The authors of the report cautioned investigators to consider this possible interaction in analysis of studies relating the ingestion of aspirin (and similar □**drugs**□) and alcohol to a possible impact on coronary-artery disease. The study raises important questions without making grandiose claims or unjustified extrapolations.[23]

Bob could only respond with silent thoughts. The rationale is that aspirin prevents platelet aggregation—clustering of disk-shaped blood elements that are involved with blood coagulation and clotting. Test results attempting to demonstrate the aspirin/blood-clotting theory have been inconsistent.[24] One researcher suggests that much of the anti-platelet activity of aspirin may be lost before it reaches the target area as it makes its passage through the gut and liver.

Another negative factor is the aspirin-alcohol interaction and its impact on gastric mucosa, which has long been recognized.[25,26] The combination of agents that cause gastritis and can aggravate or cause gastric lesions and impair coagulation can have dire consequences, especially for anyone using these substances regularly.[27] To Bob's amazement, many of the doctors confessed that they took aspirin routinely, and recommended it to patients as a clotting preventive.

One of the seminars Bob attended presented advancements in surgical methods. Bob was fascinated by innovations made possible through today's technology. Most of the methods described were medical manipulations created to relieve symptoms and, in a few cases, to reduce risk. No one said anything at this seminar or any other about surgical intervention constituting an admission of failure of other treatment.

And of course no one said anything about food or nutrients. Bob recalled a statement made by Dr. Robert Peshek, president of *The Journal of Applied Nutrition*. Dr. Peshek interviewed colleagues who were on the staffs of universities in various parts of the country. Their common reason for not teaching nutrition is that they do not know where to begin. Universities are not ready for nutrition. But nutrition has been ready—since the birth of humans.[28]

Another seminar discussed "patient compliance." The very term disturbs Bob. Compliance is "the act or process of conforming or adapting one's actions to someone else's desires or demands." This hardly suggests a physician-patient relationship that is built on trust and confidence. Are compassion and human values in medicine a thing of the past? Is it possible to maintain these values when medical practice is described as a "business"; delivering medical care is described as "producing a product"; human interactions are increasingly described in terms of *financial transactions?*[29]

There was much emphasis on techniques to increase the absorbability of □**drugs**□. Patches and pumps attached to the patient are being developed to tie in chemically with the patient's blood. The goal is to release the drug when needed. Bob sees this as good news and bad news: good for those who need it, but unfortunate for those who might heal without the drug. (The greater the absorption, the greater the risk of side effects.) And most unfortunate that some of this money is not going in the direction of *prevention,* in which case the need for drugs would be diminished.

Bob picked up a copy of *The International Journal of Biosocial Research,* attempting once again to read. His eye caught this passage:

After forty years as a student and practitioner of medicine I have reluctantly concluded that much of what I have done has been a waste of time. The world is little better off and may soon be worse off than in my student days. I believe this is so because medicine—by which I mean the whole art and science of improving and preserving health, and not just that part of it performed by doctors of medicine—is on the wrong track . . . We are heading for disaster if we keep on. That is my view.

This eloquent statement was written by Sam McClatchie, M.D., and labeled, "Misdirected Medicine."[30]

The most valuable information of the trip came from his plane companion, the little old lady sitting on his right. As dinner was being served homeward bound, she was handed a special meal. It was fruit, fresh fruit! "All you have to do is ask for it," she explained. "Every airline offers the option of a fresh fruit platter." Perhaps it was not exactly a "balanced" meal, but it was real food, nothing dismembered, nothing like the vegetarian atrocity.

The gentleman on his left laid out several bottles of prescription medicines. As Bob watched the meticulous arrangement of the nostrums, a two-line verse kept going round in his head:

He used to dine not wisely, but too well: hence all his ills;
And there is nothing now agrees with him, excepting pills.

BEN'S DINNER COMPANY

To BHT Or Not To BHT

"It used to take a lot more onions to smother a five-dollar steak," thought Ben, as he carried his dinner platter in to the TV room, which was a small comfortable area where he enjoyed most of his meals. He had the best of both worlds: he dined at home when he wanted entertainment, debates, and "canned" soap operas. He took his meals at the Senior Citizens' Club when he wanted entertainment, debates, and "live" soap operas.

Checking the *TV Guide,* Ben was delighted to see that he was in time for the start of a panel discussion on the antioxidant, butylated hydroxytoluene (BHT). His interest in the subject had been piqued when he listened to his granddaughter and grandson debating the issue at last Sunday's family get-together.

The three adversaries on the program were: an author/researcher, a professor of biochemistry, and a medical doctor. Ben started his meal just as the discussion got under way.

Author: "The free radical theory of aging is becoming widely accepted. This theory proposes that aging can be looked upon as a result of continuous 'internal radiation.' Radiation causes its damage by creating dangerous, highly reactive chemicals called free radicals. There are substances called free radical quenchers, which keep free radicals under control. One of these is the antioxidant BHT."

Doctor: "No one has ever proved that you can increase life-span of primates using antioxidants. Do you know of any tests showing that BHT prolongs life? Where are your double-blind studies? Where are the controls?"

Professor: "I don't think we are questioning the premise itself. The antioxidant properties of BHT can retard the aging process in accordance with the free radical theory. What we don't fully understand is the mechanism of how this works. It may protect against the loss of some as yet unidentified *dietary* factor or it may improve the efficiency in the *nutrient-metabolism-utilization* process.[31]

Author: "If scientific proof is the only convincing argument the doctor will accept, I can offer specifics. Dr. Denham Harman, originator of the free radical theory, has extended the life-span of mice.[32] A large number of similar studies have been documented. This antioxidant also provides some degree of protection from environmental cancer. It acts in a chemopreventive fashion."

Professor: "But although it does lessen the toxicity and carcinogenicity of some chemicals and physical agents, it potentiates the toxicity and carcinogenicity of others. It has definitely promoted the occurrence of chemically induced cancers. There is a vast complexity of interrelationships here.[33] You can't simplify these relationships, or you lose the essence."

Author: "The American Cancer Society has granted almost a million dollars for research on the anticancer properties of BHA, which is very similar to BHT."

Doctor: "Several studies have shown that BHT may be a behavioral teratogen. A teratogen is a substance causing malformation of the fetus. Chronic ingestion by pregnant mice and eventually by their offspring results in decreased sleeping, increased social and isolation induced aggression, and severe learning deficits.[34,35] Since BHT abounds in our foods (as an additive), I wonder if the current profusion of antisocial behavior in children and young adults today may be BHT-related."

Author: "Adding BHT to your food is protecting you. Ground meats such as hamburgers, hot dogs, and sausages place you at risk. The grinding process, the addition of extra fat, and many other □process-ing□ techniques create the problem.[36] I would not want to purchase meat without BHT, or some other potent antioxidant, because these foods are particularly subject to □peroxidation□. The BHT (or other antioxidant) acts as the stronghold, or 'coat of mail,' against attack. Electrons are like glue, which hold molecules together. Oxidants grab electrons interfering with the glue. When enough electrons are 'stolen,' the molecule falls apart. This is a very general interpretation of the peroxidation process.[37] Well, I don't want my molecules falling apart."

Professor: " I would like to see more widespread use of *natural* antioxidants in those foods—antioxidants such as ☆**vitamin C**☆ and ☆**vitamin E**☆ and the ☆**trace element**☆ selenium, and dimethylglycine (known as B_{15}). My body already knows how to metabolize and degrade these antioxidants. It learned how millions of years ago. I'm afraid new chemical antioxidants will shut down *necessary* oxidative functions as well as unnecessary functions."

Doctor: "Besides, BHT accumulates in body fat. It's a good example of needless use of synthetic food additives."[38]

Author: "The FDA has sanctioned the use of BHT as an additive by placing it on its GRAS list—the list of products *generally regarded as safe.*"

Professor: "Maybe the GRAS is not always greener. Other items have been gold-starred for this list, and were stricken from it years later because they turned out to be deleterious—Red Dye #2, Cyclamates, Kepone, among many."

Doctor: "BHT is a highly reactive product. Several of my patients and those of my colleagues have been taking it orally (against our better judgment) and we have seen:

worsening of rhinitis (inflammation of nasal mucous membrane)
asthmatic flare-ups within five to sixty minutes of ingestion

profuse perspiration
suffusion of the conjunctiva in the eye
skin blisters and eye hemorrhaging[39]
headache
pain high in the back of the sternal bone and radiating to the back
flushing
hives in patients with skin problems[40]."

Author: "Taking BHT is experimental. People should be aware of that. And there may be some people who are supersensitive. These people should not take BHT, and should read labels carefully."

Professor: "Reading labels gives no assurance that BHT will be avoided. BHT could be incorporated in food packaging, or in animal feeds. There are secondary ingredients, which often carry BHT. These are not necessarily on the label.[41] And the ingredient could appear under an alias, such as 'freshness preserver.'

"It is almost impossible to buy a ▢**processed**▢ food product that is devoid of BHT or its close cousin, BHA. It appears in nutmeats, raisins, milk, candied fruit, whipped topping mixes, imitation fruit drinks, breakfast foods, extracts, spices, even pet foods."

Doctor: "It causes histological changes in brain tissues."[42,43]

Professor: "It is part of food-packaging paper; waxed paper; milk carton containers; potato chip, cereal, and cookie containers; bread, butter, and cheese wrappers—even rubber gaskets that seal food jars."

Author: "If you knew that BHT could cure your hangover, would you take it? Well, it does cure hangovers."

Doctor: "If BHT and alcohol are taken together in large doses, a synergistic effect usually takes place: the clearance of alcohol from your liver may be slowed down. You won't have a headache hangover, but your liver will be 'hung over.' "[44]

Professor: "And it's even found in chewing gum. And in mashed potatoes."

Doctor: "At highest risk to BHT intoxication are: individuals with cardiovascular disease; vitamin K deficiency; hepatic disease, including abnormalities in fat metabolism; pulmonary disease; renal disorders; intestinal disorders. Women of child-bearing age should avoid any concentration of BHT. Who's left?"[45]

Professor: "—animal fats: bacon, chicken fat, butter, cream, shortenings; ▢**fried foods**▢ like potato chips, doughnuts."

Author: "The fats and oils containing such antioxidant preservatives are far safer than unprotected fats and oils."

Doctor: "We are misplacing our emphasis. Let's work on the fats and oils. Why can't these commodities be safe, and fresh, and not rancid? We all know that chemicals with low molecular weights are likely to cause bodily reactions because they are broken down and absorbed quickly. BHT has a low molecular weight."

Professor: "—baked goods of all kinds, including candies and crackers and cookies; □processed□ meats and fish; salad oils and salad dressings."[46]

Doctor: "BHT has been shown to increase the rate of urinary excretion of ☆**ascorbic acid**☆ and to elevate serum cholesterol."[47]

Professor: "—cosmetics, drugs, gelatin desserts."

Author: "BHT added to gasoline can solve the problem of gummed-up carburetors that make it difficult to start engines of lawn mowers, pleasure boats, campers, trail bikes, and generators. And it can help humans in the same way."[48]

Doctor: "Unfortunately, most of the tests have been conducted with rats. It has been shown that BHT accumulates in fat tissues of humans in greater concentrations than it does in test animals.[49] We still do not have controlled studies of humans."

Author: "But we do know that free radicals cause age pigment accumulation that slowly chokes brain cells to death and results in brownish 'age spots' in your skin."[50]

Doctor: "Several countries have banned BHT completely."

Author: "BHT can prevent the symptoms of herpes from surfacing. Professor, have you run out of foods containing BHT?"

Professor: "Unfortunately, no. But I'd like to discuss another aspect. A living cell of a human being is in an ecological balance. There are nutrients and antioxidants participating and supporting the survival of the cell all the time.

"Of course the oxidative processes are dangerous. So is too much glucose, but you couldn't exist without it. These processes take place under very tightly controlled circumstances. Your cell has the ability to take the hand of an oxygen molecule and guide it to where it is supposed to go, and let it do whatever it is supposed to do. And that is the function of the antioxidants—to control that reactivity."

Author: "But our diet today is producing too many free radicals. We need to increase the National Guard."

Professor: "If there is oxidative damage, it is because something is happening in the wrong place at the wrong time."

Author: "You had a doughnut before we went on the air. How would you protect yourself against the rancidity of the fat in that doughnut? You do agree that there was probably □rancid fat□ in that doughnut?"

Professor: "Of course. But there are hundreds of natural antioxidant combinations. All you have to do is supply the basic natural raw materials."

Author: "That's what I'm doing when I take BHT."

Professor: "I said *natural* raw materials. BHT is derived from petroleum. BHT is nonspecific, and can interfere with important oxidative processes needed for detoxification, plus other normal cellular functions. The fact is that it does have an effect on the liver. This indicates to me that it is preventing that vital organ from working at peak efficiency. The only place I would use BHT is in my gas tank. Everyone knows that ☆vitamin C☆ and ☆vitamin E☆ are antioxidants, because they have been studied so much, but there are many other antioxidants. I consume foods that contain ☆trace elements☆ like selenium, iron, calcium, zinc. These participate in antioxidant steps.

"Many spices, herbs, and flavorings—such as cloves, oregano, sage, rosemary, and vanilla—are antioxidants.

"You cannot always *piecemeal* nutrition. You run the risk of getting in the way of your own body requirements for oxidation. When will we learn that we cannot interfere with basic cell function?"

Doctor: "If you dump chemicals into a lake, is it polluted? You can't answer that unless you know how big the lake is, and what else is in the lake. I agree with the professor. There is too much BHT around. You don't know if something is safe until it is tested with a very controlled protocol."

Professor: "While you, dear author, *experiment,* and you, good doctor, wait for the *controlled studies,* I know what I have to do, not only for longevity, but also for life *quality.* I consume foods that are ☆nutrient-dense☆, foods that have a profusion of ☆vitamins☆ and ☆minerals☆, which in turn serve as catalysts for ☆enzymes☆. Enzymes enable cells to carry out their myriad functions, including oxidative processes. And, of course, I minimize my intake of □rancid foods□. I rarely eat any bottled salad dressings, or commercially fried products. How many rivets can we remove from the airplane wing before it falls off?"

"Well," thought Ben, "my cells must know how to make mincemeat out of those □free radicals□. I like the professor's views. He doesn't want to be a guinea pig. I don't have time to wait for the studies. It's real food that tramples those free varmints into the dust. And maybe real food doesn't have too many of those destroyers to begin with.

"We ask a lawyer for legal advice. We ask the accountant to go over our business records. Why don't they ask an old-timer about aging? After all, who else remembers when a juvenile delinquent was a kid with an overdue library book? Who else remembers when you saved money for a rainy day instead of April 15? Or when we didn't have to □defrost□ food before we ate it? I've been around a long time. I can tell them a thing or two."

MIKE AND MEG AND GETTING FRESH

Mike Without His Hat

Meg and Mike were not dining in a dimly lit restaurant. There was no linen cloth on the table. An empty Perrier bottle with a single rose served as centerpiece. But the menu could not have been more outstanding.

When Meg accepted Mike's dinner invitation, he warned her it would not be a run-of-the-mill meal. Meg was delighted to be taken to *Getting Fresh,* one of the best natural food restaurants in the city.

By the time they were seated, they knew a great deal about each other. The discovery of a major common goal created an especially jubilant bond between them: each was on a diet improvement campaign for different reasons, but the recommended food additions and deletions were the same.

There were so many enticements on the menu, they agreed to order different items and share.

THE APPETIZER:
Hummus on rice cakes for Meg; Greek broccoli for Mike

Hummus on Rice Cakes

Hummus is a popular Syrian or Turkish appetizer, most often served at parties or restaurants rather than with everyday home meals. One wonders if the Middle East cultures have always known what our medical journals are currently proving with double-blind studies—that ☆whole foods☆ are more healthful than foods which have had their natural architecture changed. Among the research demonstrating this:

- The Royal Infirmary in Bristol, England, studied the effects of in-gesting apples, applesauce, and apple juice. The results: An apple is digested more than ten times faster in the form of extracted ap-ple juice than when it is contained within the fibrous architecture of a whole apple. In the form of applesauce, it is assimilated nearly three times faster. These findings confirm that the natural fiber of the whole apple slows the ingestion of nutrients. (Slower inges-tion is more efficient.) The whole apple also confers extra satiety, suggesting that satiety may be partly dependent on the need to chew fiber. What is surprising is that the body handles different forms of an apple differently, not only when fiber is removed, as in apple juice, but also when fiber has merely been physically disrupted, as in applesauce. In preparing the applesauce for the study, nothing was added; nothing was taken away. Simply because you are not chewing the apple, your body responds differently.

There are other differences, too, including variations in rates of insulin release, and in each case the effects are more negative as the distortion of the original form of the apple increases.[51]

- Less fat absorption occurs after the ingestion of peanut butter than after that of peanut oil, with still lower fat absorption when eating the whole peanut. The more processing the peanut undergoes, the greater the hyperabsorption of fat when ingested. (Peanut oil has actually been shown to cause the most arterial damage of several vegetable oils tested in primate studies.)[52,53]
- Wholemeal bread produces a greater feeling of satiety than white bread. In research examining bread varieties, volunteers were asked to eat bread to a point of comfortable fullness. Increased quan-tities of white bread were consumed compared with the whole grain before satiety was reached.[54]
- Rice slurry causes a more rapid rise in blood glucose (sugar) than whole rice grains. The rapid rise, of course, is less desirable. The more homogenized the food, the more rapid the rise in blood glu-cose.[55]

Although Middle Eastern people of long ago did not know about fluctuating blood glucose levels or other functional reactions to spe-cific food products, the wisdom of the ages dictated the custom of serving hummus only on special occasions. The tradition is ongoing even to-day.

The ingredients comprising hummus are exceedingly healthful.

Hummus is made with pounded chick-peas (known as garbanzo beans), sesame seed paste (known as tahini), and seasonings. The addition of the seeds to the beans elevates the dish to one of complete protein. The chick-pea is to hummus as the apple is to applesauce—in terms of the architectural change of the whole food.

Chick-peas are loaded with great nutrients. Their yield of protein per cultivated acre is higher than any other ☆**leguminous**☆ grain, with the exception of peanuts.[56] They have a respectable ☆**calcium**☆ content, and contain a significant amount of iron, among other important nutrients.

A researcher at New York University Medical Center has shown that a substance known as protease inhibitor, which is found almost entirely in ☆**vegetables**☆, can prevent cancer in test animals. The valuable protease inhibitor is present in chick-peas and other ☆**legumes**☆.[57]

And besides, chick-peas are delicious. In many European countries, they are served in stews, soups, and salads. Meg commented that she had learned to ☆**sprout**☆ chick-peas, a very simple process. She, like the Europeans, adds them to salads. "They're rather bland, but crunchy, so they add texture."

Sesame seeds are also high in protein. One of the great values of sesame is its unique amino acid composition. Sesame seeds contain methionine and tryptophan, amino acids missing from most other vegetable protein sources, such as soy bean, wheat, peas, seeds, and buckwheat.[58] Every body cell requires methionine. When the body has its saturation of methionine, the excess is converted to choline, a nutrient usually on the "wanted" list. Choline aids in the ability to handle cholesterol, and also helps the process by which the body produces energy instead of fat.[59] Tryptophan is important for skin and hair health. It is also the precursor of niacin, thereby taking on the responsibility of providing a good nervous system.[60]

The oil of sesame seeds is famous for its resistance to ▢**rancidity**▢. Unlike most seeds, they contain a greater ratio of ☆**calcium**☆ to phosphorus, which is desirable. The seeds lend a delicious nutlike flavor.

When it was said that good things come in small packages, the sesame seed must have been considered. The minute seed is one of the most digestible and alkaline protein foods known. In ancient Babylon, women ate halvah (a sesame and honey mixture) to restore vitality and sex appeal. Roman soldiers who swept through Europe survived on limited rations, which included sesame seeds.

Garlic, lemon juice, olive oil, tamari (soy sauce), with trimmings of parsley and mint complete the hummus recipe.

Both Meg and Mike were making every effort to stay away from wheat products. This is no easy task because wheat products are found in: pancakes, waffles, breads, cookies, crackers, cakes, breaded foods, pasta, bouillon cubes, chocolate candy, cooked mixed meat dishes, ice-cream cones, most cooked sausages, thickenings in ice cream, anything with gluten, and the coatings of many fried foods. Rye products often contain wheat, as do most of the commercial cold cereals and flour mixtures.[61]

They were so pleased that *Getting Fresh,* aware of the growing recognition of wheat sensitivity, offers alternatives such as rice cakes and other crackers made of gluten-free grains (millet and buckwheat). Hummus spread on rice cakes is a delectable appetizer.

Greek Broccoli

Broccoli stalks, buds, and leaves are lightly simmered with lemon, onion, tomatoes, and basil. The seasonings endow this preparation with an air of Greece. And the broccoli endows the eater with an anticancer food, according to the American Cancer Society. The effects of environmental carcinogens are reduced by eating cabbage, cauliflower, brussel sprouts, and broccoli.[62] Their inhibiting power has been demonstrated for mammary and gastric cancer. It is believed that these foods induce an effect on an ☆**enzyme**☆ present in high concentration in many tissues—an enzyme that has the ability to break down carcinogens.[63,64]

Broccoli is also a major source of vitamin K. Note the levels of vitamin K in an average portion (100 grams) of these vegetables:[65]

Turnip greens	650 mgs
Broccoli	200
Lettuce	129
Cabbage	125
Spinach	89
Green beans	14
Potatoes	3

Mike and Meg talked about their attitudes toward meat, and how hard it was—not so long ago—to imagine a meal without it. Most people of the world, however, don't eat much meat. They get protein from grains, ☆**vegetables**☆, ☆**legumes**☆, fruits, nuts, and ☆**seeds**☆. Although the United States makes up about 7 percent of the world's population, we consume 30 percent of total animal protein.

Mike offered this bit of trivia: "The first notable American vegetarian was the printer, statesman, inventor, and writer, Ben Franklin."[66]

THE SALAD:
Cauliflower pecan salad for Meg, with mustard-horseradish dressing; sunshine carrot salad for Mike with curry dressing; marinated cucumbers and marinated mushrooms

Cauliflower Pecan Salad

Mark Twain called cauliflower "cabbage with a college education," and he didn't even know about its anticancer qualities. The cancer protection may be because of its large amount of ☆**vitamin A**☆ and ☆**vitamin C**☆. There is so much vitamin C in cauliflower, some of it is still retained even after cooking. Raw cauliflower adds crunchiness.

A major ingredient of each salad was shredded carrot. The association of beta-carotene as an anticancer agent is now well known. Many reports which have appeared in the last decade show that retinol (the form of vitamin A found in mammals) is effective in inhibiting cancer in experimental animals.[67] More recently attention has been focused on studies showing an inverse correlation between blood retinol levels and cancer risk in humans. Dietary intake of ☆**vitamin A**☆ lowers the prospect of cancer—especially cancer of the lung and oral and gastrointestinal tract.[68,69,70] (Of interest, however, is the lack of effect on cancer risk in women using ▫**oral contraceptives**▫. Despite higher than average blood retinol levels, their cancer incidence is not reduced.[71,72])

It is nutritionally advantageous that fresh carrots are available all year. Meg provided these minutiae: "The ancient Greeks used carrots as a remedy for venereal disease; the Arabs considered it an aphrodisiac." (The reasoning was that the vegetable's shape provided a clue to which part of the body would be helped by it.)

In early Celtic literature, the carrot was referred to as "honey underground." With the exception of the beet, it is the sweetest vegetable. Even though its sugar content is 10 to 15 percent, it is a ☆**low-calorie food**☆ (about forty-two calories per 100 grams). Darker carrots contain a greater amount of carotene.[73]

There were bits of red and green pepper weaving through the carrot and cauliflower. As green pepper continues to grow, its color shifts. Vibrant red peppers are more mature and sweeter, and have more ☆**vitamin C**☆. (It has been said that adding red peppers to a salad is like sending it to Hawaii for a two-week vacation.)

Vitamin C is one of the most unstable nutrients. It is sensitive to heat, oxygen, and the presence of toxic minerals. Even storage in polyethylene containers hastens its destruction. Meg and Mike conjectured that the chefs at *Getting Fresh* must know the importance of raw foods, and the fragility of vitamin C—the salads were so huge!

The therapeutic activities of vitamin C are profuse:

- A high vitamin C intake is associated with an increased detoxifying ability of the liver.[74]
- Remember the mighty mitochondria? Vitamin C is necessary for the transport of fatty acids into mitochondria (that important energy substrate in the muscle cells.)[75]
- Vitamin C is necessary to maintain integrity of connective tissues, because ascorbate is required for collagen synthesis.
- Total cholesterol and triglycerides are highest in test animals with a marginal deficiency of vitamin C, and lowest in vitamin C saturated animals.[76] There is a negative correlation between vitamin C status and cholesterol, but a positive relationship between vitamin C and high-density lipoproteins—the good guy cholesterol factions.[77]
- With an increasing level of vitamin C in the liver, there is an increase in the proportion of animals in which no gallstones form.[78]
- Vitamin C increases the intestinal uptake and metabolism of iron.[79]
- Vitamin C quenches □**free radicals**□, labeled as the major cause of aging.[80]
- There is a protective effect of vitamin C in severe allergic reactions due to its ability to lower histamine concentrations.[81]
- Ascorbic acid is reported to be protective against viruses, including measles, mumps, herpes zoster, and respiratory viruses.[82,83,84]

Meg confessed that pecan pie is her favorite of all foods. But she was quite content to settle for a handful of pecans dotting the salad. Having read that Dr. John Ellis (known for his nutritional cures) advocates twelve raw pecans a day for relieving some forms of painful neuritis and arthritis, Meg bemoaned the fact that she suffered from acne, and not arthritis. Dr. Ellis believes the relief is due to the high vitamin B_6 content of pecans.[85] Heating significantly decreases the bioavailability of B_6, and most of the foods that contain the vitamin are usually cooked: ☆liver☆, kidney, heart, milk, ☆eggs☆, beef, whole grains. ▫Heating▫ also affects the *quality* of the vitamin.[86] It is, however, also found in ☆brewer's yeast☆, cantaloupe, and cabbage. This is indeed a high B_6 salad!

Since Native Americans gathered pecans for use as a staple food, it obviously has a range of sustaining nutrients. A nut "milk" was extracted from pecans by the Indians, and this was used as gruel in making corncakes.

Mustard-Horseradish Dressing

As people become involved in healthful gourmet cooking, more attention is paid to the wonderful herbs and seasonings available. Using condiments has become a lost art in the average American household, where almost all foods are doused with cascades of salt, or perhaps swim in that sugary red deception called ketchup. (Ketchup has a higher sugar content than most ice cream!)

Not only do ☆herbs☆ and spices add a range of flavors to foods, but they are nutrient laden products. The chefs of India have learned to embellish dishes with herbs which aid digestion or curtail flatulence.[87]

Over the centuries, herbs have been used medicinally, both internally and topically. Meg's mother told her that *her* grandmother poured hot water over bruised mustard seeds to create a soothing bath for tired feet. Grated fresh horseradish was applied to aching joints. Meg's great grandmother would look askance at any medicament that she could not eat—even if applied to the surface of her body.

Mustard is a condiment second only to salt and pepper in popularity. In very early times it was the custom to chew tiny mustard seeds with meat. Even the Romans prepared a mustard sauce. They also used it medically as a warming poultice in obstinate cases of pneumonia or bronchitis, and for victims of poisoning or upset stomach.[88]

Many of today's commercial brands of mustard are fine products, devoid of sugar and additives. When preparing mustard dressings, horseradish is often added to strengthen the taste. Since the flavor of horseradish is lost in cooking, it is always used raw. Horseradish is a good source of the ☆**minerals**☆ potassium and calcium.

Sunshine Carrot Salad

Among other goodies, sunshine carrot salad boasts of sunflower seeds. The Russians, knowing the great value of this superior food, use sunflower seeds extensively. In addition to their pectin content (a detoxifying substance), sunflower seeds have just the right kind of essential fatty acids, hard come by in the average diet. Meg's recent understanding of the relationship between essential fatty acids and skin problems is the reason why she always has a packet of sunflower seeds in her purse.

Meg's nutrition counselor advised that she purchase sunflower seeds *in the shell,* unroasted and unsalted. Roasting destroys nutrients. The sunflower seed contains a living growth factor. When the seed is planted, it produces a huge amount of plant growth and more than a thousand seeds. Cook it, and it's dead—it will not produce anything. When adding to salads, grains, and sandwich spreads, it is impractical to buy the seeds in the shell. For use as embellishment, Meg purchases shelled sunflower seeds, and sprouts them one or two days. This multiplies nutrient value, and compensates for any rancidity.

Another addition to this salad is freshly grated coconut. It is difficult to find coconut which does not have sugar and other additives (propylene glycol, BHT, and BHA), unless the source is a natural food outlet. Or unless whole coconuts are purchased, and they are shredded at home.

It is obvious that *Getting Fresh* has done its own coconut shredding. The brown skin that clings so tightly to the white meat has been left intact: that's where most of the coconut's important food elements have been concentrated.

Because coconuts grow on beaches close to the sea, they are rich in minerals often lacking in land-grown seeds. In tropical countries the coconut has the reputation of helping disorders of the liver and stomach.

Curry Dressing

In India, curry powder is not usually bought as a blend. When the cook does the blending, the strength and flavor of a curry dish varies in infinite ways. *Getting Fresh* uses freshly blended curry in all recipes, despite the fact that only dry leaves are available in the marketplace in this country. (They have a private source.) Fresh curry leaves provide a highly aromatic flavor. In too many restaurants, curry is used as a veil for leftovers. Never at *Getting Fresh.*

Marinated Cucumbers and Marinated Mushrooms

Benzoate of soda, sulphur dioxide, calcium chloride, polysorbate 80, FD & C Yellow #5, xanthine gum, alum. No, these are not listings of a tire patch cement formula. This is what you are probably eating when you swallow your food with pickles, relish, or sauerkraut, ◻**commercially**◻ prepared. Sweetening agents, such as corn syrup, are also used.

These chemicals are not necessary for creating spicy, delicious pickled foods. At *Getting Fresh,* the cucumbers are marinated in cider vinegar and seasonings, and the mushrooms in unrefined olive oil with spices and herbs.

ENTREE:
Tamale pie for Meg; egg foo yung with rice almondine for Mike

Tamale Pie

"Full of beans." "He spilled the beans." "She doesn't know beans about that." "He's skinny as a beanpole." "Use your bean." "It's not worth a hill of beans." Just as the word ☆**bean**☆ in vocabulary can be negative or positive, so the bean itself has been favored and disfavored over the centuries. Historians declare that the ancient Egyptians dedicated temples to beans, worshipping them as symbols of life itself. The Romans gambled with beans, and Scottish witches were said to take their moonlight rides on beanstalks instead of broomsticks.

Today, beans are for eating. You have probably seen round, flat, little, big, white, black, green, red, spotted, dotted, fresh, and dry beans. But sometimes there is confusion about what a bean is or isn't. ☆**Legumes**☆ belong to the family of plants bearing their seeds in pods. A legume is an oblong pod. Beans are legumes, but so are peas. So are lentils, and many other plants, including peanuts. Peas and beans are variations on a theme. Just as a Doberman pinscher and a westy white terrier are both dogs, beans and peas and lentils are all legumes.

Whatever the genus or species, most beans are nutritious and in-expensive, but are considered low status in our country. Too many people think that because beans are a hearty staple, they belong to an era long gone. What a mistake! Beans are rich in high quality protein, ☆**low in fat**☆, have fiber and important ☆**minerals**☆, plus a good so-dium/potassium ratio:

In One Average Portion of Beans

Protein	8.9 grams	A lot! That's good.
Fat	0.5 grams	Very little! That's good.
Carbohydrates	25.2 grams	Not bad!
Calcium	57.0 milligrams	Enough to count!
Sodium/potassium ratio		Excellent! (more po-tassium than so-dium)
B vitamins		A small amount, but enough!

Usually, the seeds of the pod are eaten. One exception to this is the green bean, in which case the pod itself is eaten. The seeds inside the green bean never develop to any significant size. Because green beans are not mature, they have a different nutritional value than dried beans. They contain only 2 percent protein, 3 percent carbohydrates, and only about 18 calories in a hundred grams. (Just a reminder—a hundred grams is about an average portion or fistful.)

No refrigeration is needed for long storage of any dried beans. They are almost nonperishable. Beans are so versatile, they can be boiled, baked, fried, sprouted, flaked, ground into flour, or cooked whole. Americans are, we're glad to say, beginning to have more respect for beans. They are the basis for cuisine—from simple to elegant—the world over.

In every culture, beans are served with another food that is com-plementary in terms of protein. "Protein complementarity" was never stated in scientific terms. The scientific understanding is relatively new. But the knowledge that these combinations engendered good health is as old as time.[89]

Beans are a basic, easily available product—a direct food crop that can be transformed into many healthful, beautiful, and exciting treats. Tamale pie, which uses pinto beans as its base, is such an example.

In addition to sprouting chick-peas, Meg said she sprouts mung and adzuki beans. Mike was familiar with mung beans, but had never heard of adzuki. Meg made Mike's mouth water as she described them, and explained how they enhance her homemade salads (which she promised to prepare for Mike soon).

Egg Foo Yung with Rice Almondine

Egg foo yung is tastefully cooked with ☆**eggs**☆, ☆**sprouts**☆, mushrooms, celery, and grated onion. Whole almonds (not blanched) are added to brown rice and baked with tamari and other seasonings.

Meg and Mike each knew something their friends, and in some cases, their friends' physicians, did not seem to be aware of: *There is no relationship between egg intake and coronary heart disease incidence. Egg consumption is unrelated to blood cholesterol levels.*[90,91,92,93,94,95]

In early times people traveled to mineral springs or spas to drink sulfur water. This sulfur elixir is found in eggs. Misguided warnings against egg eating may result in sulfur deficiency in many people.[96] Onions and garlic contain an appreciable amount of sulfur too. (The tear gas from sliced onions is a simple sulfur compound, and the smell of garlic is characteristic of organic sulfur.)

Their friends (and again, their friends' physicians) are just as confused about grains as they are about eggs. But then not so long ago, Meg and Mike would have missed their way with grains too. In fact, Meg, when tasting her first bowl of millet, said, "I like this kind of oatmeal." She knows better now.

Basically, a grain is a seed, and is made up of three parts: the germ, which will, upon germination and sprouting, give rise to the first tiny leaves and rootlets; the endosperm, or starchy bulk of the grain, which nourishes the seedling during its early growth; and the bran or tough outer covering which protects the grain. As long as the grain or seed remains intact, it will live for some time in a dormant condition. It has been reported that grains found in Egyptian tombs have actually sprouted.

Whole grains are a major part of almost every culture's diet. The Orientals eat a lot of rice. Mexicans eat beans, corn, and rice in many different forms. In Europe, it's rye. The Russians eat buckwheat (kasha) as a staple food. In Africa and many other areas, millet is the important grain.

But Americans eat virtually no *whole* grains, even though the United States is one of the largest grain producers in the world. Grain cookery in general is unfamiliar to most Americans, who, if they purchase grains at all, buy them in "instant" preparations, or as milled varieties—rarely ever intact. The nutrition of the grain is disrupted when the grain is ground, cracked, or rolled. It is no longer "alive."

Patterns of grain eating developed independently in all parts of the world, combining cooked grains with other products to form complete protein meals. The patterns endured because they worked so well. Grains can be prepared with straight-out simplicity (cooked with some liquid and served as a porridge), or elevated to a cuisine that rivals the most artful of edibles.[97]

All cereal grains can be baked into bread. During imperial times in ancient Rome, each citizen was entitled to free grain from the public dole, as well as free public entertainment. This policy was summed up in the terse slogan, "Bread and Circuses."[98] Our modern-day cliché, "Bread: The Staff of Life," is no longer the valid message it once was. Most of our bread is so denatured, the saying has been paraphrased: "Bread: The *Strife* of Life."

Rice is probably the world's most single important food. Only the tough outer husk is stripped to yield whole or brown rice, but most of the bran and embryo are removed to produce white rice. White rice is washed, cleaned, and polished. A further step is "coating," which adds a layer of corn syrup and talc to give it a pearly luster. (Corn is high on the list of common allergens. Anyone sensitive to white rice may in fact be responding to the corn coating.) Rice that proceeds beyond the first step of milling loses ☆**nutrients**☆, including most of its ☆**vitamin B**☆, fat, and some of its protein. Brown rice is easily digested, nourishing, and very palatable.[99]

The almonds gilding the baked rice dish are among the most popular of edible nuts. Almonds are about 50 percent oil and 15 percent protein, with significant quantities of vitamin B_1, ☆**calcium**☆, iron, and phosphorus. In Spain and Portugal, sweet almond oil is preferred in the kitchen for frying fish and vegetables. The almond, by the way, is a cousin of the peach.

Nuts in general have more ☆**food value per weight**☆ than meat, grains, or fruit. Early food chemists called nut protein "vegetable casein" because of its close resemblance to the protein of milk.

Mike confessed he was surprised that he was not finding it painful to give up old favorites. In fact, some of those foods upset his stomach now. Meg suggested that his diet probably wasn't all that bad to begin with. "If you had to give up drugs like □**caffeine**□ or □**nicotine**□ or lots of □**sugar**□, you would have experienced withdrawal symptoms for awhile. And you probably would be craving those foods now."

They talked about trying to make sandwiches without bread, and ice cream without milk, about finding something to put on granola, and about raising resistance by eating before going to cocktail parties.

As they were parting, Meg commented with a pleasant smile, "I never saw you without your blue cap before."

Mike responded with his own vibrant smile, "Were you surprised?"

Meg didn't answer his question, but said, "You never look untidy. Bald is neat!"

"I hope neatness counts."

"Sure it does."

SALLY'S PIT STOP

Fast Food Saves

With empty stomach but full heart, Sally emerged from the plastic surgeon's office. Her preop visit went well. She joyfully envisioned herself a month from now, *sans* under-eye folds and facial brown spots. The wait at the doctor's office had been a long one, and she was famished. "One of these days," she said, "I will remember to take food with me." Her blood sugar was so low she was tempted to eat the flowers sold by a vendor on the street corner. And then she saw it, an oasis in the desert: a fast food restaurant right before her eyes.

There was no hesitation, no reluctance. "If I must, I must." I have no choice. As Sally entered the restaurant, she thought of the innumerable meals she had eaten in such places over the years. Who ever thought of food *quality* in those days? When the family discussed dining out for the evening, her daughter would comment, "We're no different than the hunter-gatherer of long ago. We hunt for our feeding place, and we gather its food. Only we have different dangers: we may have to wait in line; or maybe they're out of chocolate ice cream just when it's our turn; the waiter may be rude; service slow. Or maybe if you're eating home you have to spend too much time preparing the food."

The Salad Bar

Sally knew her selections today would not be a choice between good and bad, but rather between bad and worse. With this thought in mind, she headed for the salad bar, where she could select:

- Potassium metabisulphite, an antibrowning agent and preservative. This is frequently used on cut fruits (such as apples) and vegetables (especially celery, cucumbers, onions, peppers, and potatoes). It can destroy ☆**vitamin B**☆ and is capable of causing damage to the digestive system and other organs.[100,101] These sulphites may create new compounds in greater concentration than is normally found in foods.[102]

Sally recalled seeing a program on *Sixty Minutes* exposing sulphiting agents. They are used mainly for cosmetic purposes. The exposé came about because people reported severe asthmatic attacks following ingestion of foods that had been sprayed with this type of antibrowning agent, which is also used on shrimp and dried fruit, and in wine.[103] A population of 10 million people has about 400,000 asthmatics.[104]

- Nine lethal sprays. Head lettuce (also called iceberg lettuce) outsells all other varieties in the country, and is the least nutritious. Head lettuce is bred and groomed for ease of packing, shipping, and storing. Sometimes as many as nine doses of "embalmers" are employed.[105]
- Heated salads. Salads such as three-bean, tuna, chicken, and so on, are often delivered to restaurants in large Number 10 cans or jars. These cans or jars are vehicles for a thermal (heating) process. The thermal process destroys ☆**enzymes**☆ to prolong shelf life. The larger the can, the longer the thermal exposure.

Heat-denatured, enzyme-deficient food places unnatural strain on enzyme-secreting organs. Changes in the weight of the pancreas and other organs have been repeatedly induced experimentally in animals by use of such diets.[106] The important provitamin A (beta-carotene) decreases as cooking time increases.[107]

Toasting bread serves as a good example of the effect of nutrient depletion which occurs during the heating process. If a slice of white bread (unenriched) is toasted for *thirty seconds*, it loses almost 10 percent of its thiamine. Whole grain bread loses 4 percent. If that same piece of bread is toasted for 70 seconds, the white bread loses more than 31 percent, and the whole grain about 21 percent of thiamine.[108]

- Cottage cheese with additives (maybe mold or slime, too!). Cottage cheese is a very fragile food product, almost as perishable as milk. Beatrice Trum Hunter (renowned consumer advocate) discusses a study in which a high count of slime and mold was found on the surface of many samples of cottage cheese. Ms. Hunter says:

Sodium hypochlorite may be used in washing the curds, which finishes the process far more quickly than the traditional bacterial one. Diacetyl may be added as a butter flavor. Objectionable amounts of salt may also be added. [A scoop of cottage cheese may have three times as much salt as a handful of salted peanuts.] Annatto or cochineal may be used as dyes, and hydrogen peroxide as a preservative. . . .

Calcium sulfate, related to plaster of Paris, is a material of questionable safety in food. It was described as a material that "hardens quickly after absorbing moisture, and its ingesting may result in obstruction, particularly at the pylorus," and "surgical relief may be necessary." . . . Calcium sulfate is permitted in cottage cheese. Mold retarders of sorbic acid, or its salts, are also permitted.[109]

- Rancid oils. It has been said that no salad oil exists that is not at least a little rancid. Most are *very* rancid. When the mechanisms of rancidity and the □processing□ steps involved in preparing these oils are thoroughly understood, the statement is more than believable.

Oxidative reactions may occur in raw materials used to express edible oils prior to □processing□.[110] The □oxidized fats□ may promote further oxidation during processing or detract from the stability of the finished product.[111,112] When the polyunsaturated fatty acid content of any food is increased, the prevention of oxidation becomes a greater problem than usual.[113]

The relation of oil or fat quality to the severity of □processing□ techniques has long been recognized. Most vegetable oils are currently obtained by solvent extraction with volatile petroleum hydrocarbons, such as hexane and acetone. These solvents are later vaporized, leaving a small residue in the oil, which the FDA regards as a safe amount. Many petroleum derivatives are known or suspected carcinogens. Does anyone really know how much is safe for everyone?[114]

Oils are also extracted by a so-called "cold" process, which is a misnomer because the extreme hydrolic pressure required to squeeze the oil out of the food raises the temperature to between 275 and 400 degrees Fahrenheit.

Removal of various associated materials (such as free fatty acids and plant gums) reduces the stability of the oil. Vital carotenes, chlorophyll, and other plant pigments are removed when the oil is treated with bleaching clay. This process involves further oxidation and ▫**free radical**▫ production.[115,116] When the product is deodorized there is a substantial reduction of essential nutrients and natural antioxidants. Despite elaborate precautions against further oxidation, additional changes occur with time.[117]

Substances added to salad dressings may be acidifiers (acetic or citric acid), antioxidants (BHT), preservatives (EDTA, potassium sorbate, sodium benzoate), thickeners (modified food starch, xanthine gum or propylene glycol alginate), flavor enhancers (MSG), crystallizing preventers (oxystearin), and emulsifiers (polysorbate 60).

Sally looked at the large containers of ▫**salad dressing**▫ sitting in tubs—out in the open—and turned away from the salad bar. Too many of the products offered here were pro-aging.

The Hot Dog

When the kids were young, and Tom washed his hot dogs down with beer, they would say, "Dad's at it again, Mom. *Frank 'n' stein.*" Ever since the family learned that 20 percent of filler meat allowed in hot dogs could be ground chicken, grain, or snout, they stopped eating franks—except on very special occasions. Another negative is the meat's sodium nitrite content. This additive can combine with secondary amines (which are organic compounds containing nitrogen) in meat or in the stomach to form nitrosamines, a group of potent carcinogens.

When the Meat Board advertised (in a medical journal, no less!) that the high sodium content of ▫**processed**▫ meats is less than that contained in processed cheese, consumer groups complained. It was pointed out that processed cheese is one of the highest sodium foods in the diet, and that the Meat Board might as well have bragged that processed meats contain less sodium than a saltshaker.[118] (The average hot dog has 500 to 625 milligrams of sodium, at least three times a person's daily need.[119])

The Hamburger

Sally grew up with the admonition never to order a hamburger in a restaurant. "It is rumored," her mother told her, "that butchers sweep sawdust from the floor of their shops into the hamburger patties, especially when the meat is intended for commercial use." (If they ever did or still do use sawdust, it could be labeled "powdered cellulose" and it might have full sanction of the FDA.)

It took Sally many years to get over her hamburger prejudice. Just when she was feeling quite comfortable consuming one, she began to get messages that the hamburger isn't, after all, the best of foods. Although she doesn't know all of the reasons for the new indictment, she would not have been surprised to learn the following:

- If an animal's carcass is not good enough to produce steaks, chops, and other cuts, it may end up in the hamburgers of one of the fast food chains.[120]
- Cages, steel bars, fluorescent lights, dusty air, and total darkness describes the environment of animals raised for mass production. Obviously this affects the quality of the final product. Jim Mason, in *Animal Factories,* says: "Today's animals are artificial to the marrow."[121]
- A feedlot steer has about three times the amount of storage-type fat as nutrient material. Compare this with a free-living animal, which has five to ten times as much nutrient material as storage fat.[122]
- A woman experienced acute symptoms of swelling of her face, trunk, and arms, plus abdominal pain. She noted that each time she had a hamburger at a well-known fast food chain, her lower lip swelled. The guilty ingredient turned out to be gum tragacanth, added to food to give bulk, thickness, and binding qualities.[123]
- Diethylstilbestrol (DES) is causally associated with cancer.[124] Consequently some governments have banned its use in meat production. This type of ▫**drug**▫ improves the live weight gain of the animal, the carcass weight, feed efficiency, and the percentage of meat yield. DES and similar drugs are not destroyed in the gut or on the first pass through the liver, so that their residues in ingested meat may have hormonal effects that can influence cancer risk if dosage is high enough.[125] Even when banned, illegal use is difficult to monitor.

The sodium content of most fast food items is much too high. These menus lack a rich source of ☆vitamin A☆. Other nutrients commonly in short supply are ☆B vitamins☆ and ☆trace elements☆, including biotin, folacin, pantothenic acid, iron, calcium, and copper. Fast food meals are excessive in calories compared with nutrients. A hamburger, □fries□, and shake total about 1,000 calories (and still no vitamin A). That same trio contains 1,240 milligrams of sodium.

The last 280 people who entered this restaurant purchased 19 shakes and 13 orders of milk, but 115 orders of □soft drinks□ and 80 cups of □coffee□.

Fast foods undergo multiple heating and cooling from the initial steps of □processing□ to the time the food is set before the customer. Here is another source for nutritional deprivation.[126,127]

Sally could not explain why she left the salad bar and settled for the thousand (or more) calories feast: a hamburger, □french fries□, and a shake. She did promise herself that it was the "last supper," that never again would she be so nutritionally indiscreet. After all, these were unusual circumstances. She was celebrating the start of a new Sally. Why was she doing it by consuming foods which had created the old Sally? Perhaps, like the rest of the world, she decided she deserved the *sweet reward,* even if this one contained more □free radicals□ than sucrose.

A dietician examining Sally's meal would have to admit that it complied with specifications of "The Four Food Groups." Dr. Ross Hume Hall, professor of biochemical nutrition, offers a "Cell's Eye View" of the Four Food Group paradigm:

This guideline devised before World War II features photographs of glasses of milk, fresh lean meat, wholesome-looking bread, fresh ☆vegetables☆ with drops of water clinging to them. This idealized view of what and how people eat no more resembles the current mainstream North American diet than the stilted mannequins in a store-front window resemble real people.

. . . From the cell's point of view, all nutrient factors are equally important and if just one is missing, the cell dies. . . . The health of a person depends on the collective health of his cells.

. . . One reason there appears to be plenty of fresh produce available is that few people eat it.[128]

The Worst of Convenience

The five worst fast food offerings were recently outlined in *Nutrition Action*, a consumer advocacy magazine, published by The Center for Science in the Public Interest. They are:

1. Wendy's Triple Cheeseburger, because of its walloping fat and sodium content. Suggested renaming: Coronary Bypass Special.
2. Extra Crispy Dark Kentucky Fried Chicken Dinner, because of its high fat and sodium content. "Extra crispy means extra fatty."
3. Burger King Whopper, because of its supplemental "special sauce," which is pure mayonnaise. "If you think the eighth-inch or less of shredded lettuce adds much nutrition, you probably believe ketchup is a vegetable."
4. Pizza Hut Super Supreme Pizza, because of its high fat and sodium content. "Forget the extras, except mushrooms or green pepper, when you eat pizza."
5. McDonald's Fillet of Fish Sandwich, because it is a fat-soaked item. "A single burger has less than half the fat."

"In several respects," says *Nutrition Action*, "fast food meals compare poorly to the meals many Americans eat at home. Few people deep fry so many foods—from chicken to potatoes to fruit pies—in a tub of beef- or lard-based fat reused many times a day."[129]

With her blood sugar level now at a comfortable level, Sally headed for the exit. As she was leaving, she saw a familiar face entering. It was the plastic surgeon's nurse. The nurse hurriedly greeted Sally, and said, "The doctor is so busy today. He hasn't even had any lunch. I'm picking up a quick dinner for him."

If the doctor isn't feeling well at the end of the day, it's because he had too many fast foods on a slow stomach.

JANE AND JIM AND GRANDPA'S BIRTHDAY

"Leave Out the MSG, Please"

"Don't forget to say, 'No MSG,' Mom. And order something with tofu. You'll like it. And not too many selections with meat. See you at seven," said Jane to her mother. Jane, Jim, and the children were getting ready to visit the grandparents, who were planning a take-out Chinese meal in celebration of Grandpa's birthday.

"You forgot to remind her to say no cornstarch and no sugar. Sometimes they'll comply with that, too," added Jim.

"Daddy, why do they use MSG if it's no good?" asked ten-year-old Jennifer.

"It makes food taste better. For that reason it's called a 'flavor enhancer.' It actually excites your taste buds."

"Can Chinese people eat MSG?"

"Good question, honey. As a matter of fact, Asians are not as sensitive to MSG as we are. There is a unique biochemical genetic metabolic difference in the way Orientals handle protein in their livers. (MSG is a protein.) The Asian liver, because it has been exposed for millennia to a low protein diet of soy and rice, is extremely efficient in managing dietary protein. So the Asian quickly converts the glutamate, and less of it is spilled into the blood after eating.[130] What I'm saying is that they have inherited the ability of their bodies to handle the MSG, and we haven't. One other problem is that MSG is derived from different sources in Eastern countries. That could contribute to difficulties, too."

"What happens if you eat it by mistake? Do you get sick?" Jennifer asked.

"Many people don't have any reactions at all. But if they do, they may feel sensations of warmth, stiffness, weakness in the limbs, tingling, pressure, headache, light-headedness, heartburn, dry mouth, or stomachaches.[131] Sometimes people get one, or a few, of these symptoms later on, or even the next day, and do not associate the problem with the Chinese meal.[132]

"One of the women in my office develops a severe asthma attack the day after eating Chinese food. Her doctor told her that the long delay between eating food containing MSG and the development of asthma is not like any other reaction to a food □additive□, and that's why she had several incidents before she was aware of what was happening.[133] Aunt Margaret gets tingling sensations in her arm from MSG, but she doesn't care. She eats the food anyway."

Jane corrected Jim. "She used to get the tingling. But she doesn't anymore—not since she found out about vitamin B_6. She takes 50 milligrams a day, and she no longer reacts to MSG."[134]

"Does that mean that anyone with a B_6 deficiency will be sensitive to MSG?" questioned Jim.

"Not necessarily. Many people with such deficiencies are not MSG reactors. It just means that, like so many other problems, there are multiple causes. The B_6, however, works for most people."

Jane continued, addressing Jennifer. "When Dad and I were babies, both grandmas fed us baby food that had MSG in it. The manufacturers put the MSG in the liver or the soup, so that when Grandma tasted the food, *she* would like it. When it was discovered that MSG not only excited taste buds, but also excited nerve endings, the baby food manufacturers agreed to eliminate it. MSG has even been shown to cause brain damage."[135]

"Mommy, if they don't use MSG in canned food anymore, why can't we eat food from cans the way my friends do?"

"Oh, it's only the baby food people who have eliminated the MSG. It's used extensively in other foods: in canned and frozen vegetables; fish fillets; soups; canned tuna; chicken à la king; soup mixes; seasonings; mayonnaise and other salad dressings; potato chips; crackers; fish sticks; franks; take-out chicken. Caterers use it because they want their food to taste the best. And you know the new sugar substitute everyone's raving about? Well, if you consume enough of that with MSG, you increase the possibility of toxic effects."[136]

Jennifer's next question was difficult to answer: "So why does our President allow it if it's so bad for us?"

Jim answered. "Well, that's a loaded question. When a famous doctor reported that MSG caused brain lesions in animals, the FDA (our government group that checks these things) requested a review. But some of the people who conducted the studies included manufacturers and food processors who use MSG in their products. When they concluded that MSG was okay, the doctor said, 'This is an industry arranged whitewash made by a group with almost no experience in neuropathology.' "[137]

"Wait a minute," interrupted Jennifer. "How come *we* used to eat all that kind of stuff?"

"We weren't as smart about nutrition as we are now. We made a mistake. We've learned that this kind of food doesn't have ☆**nutrient power**☆ because nutrients are removed before ▫**processing**▫, or because they are destroyed while they are being processed. You know what they say: you are what you eat. Do you want to be bleached and blanched, or colored and curdled? Or maybe dampened and dehydrated, emulsified, and evaporated? Maybe fried and frozen, ground and grated, heated and homogenized, mashed and molded, milled and microwaved, pasteurized and pressurized, stuffed and stored, salted and sweetened, and generally zapped?"

"Oh, Daddy, how silly."

"C'mon, you guys. Grandma and Grandpa are waiting for us with Chinese dinner. Let's go."

Grandpa's ☆Fish☆

It could have been a scene from *All in the Family*, with everyone reaching and ladling and pouring and passing and tasting and sharing the varied succulent Chinese dishes—except for Grandpa. Grandpa had a mild heart attack recently. Grandpa was eating fish.

And Grandpa was doing some good-natured complaining. "I used to brush my teeth after eating. Now I *count* my teeth after I eat. I used to pray before I eat. Now I pray after I've finished. You can't imagine what awful food Grandma is serving me. This morning I had a stack of pancakes for breakfast. I think the recipe came from Decca Records. And remember minute rice? Now it takes an hour and a quarter to prepare. Grandma used to be a cook. Now she's a direction reader. For years I paid into a plan. I expected to retire on 1200 a month. I didn't know it was going to be calories."

"Don't listen to him," Grandma said. "He's really enjoying his meals. He's even learned to do some cooking. You should taste his 'Feesh Lorraine,' and his 'Couscous' and his 'Ratatouille à la Niçoise.'"

Jane wished her father had prepared dinner this evening. His preparations sounded better than the restaurant foods they were trying to eat less of. But how do you say "no" to Grandma?

After dinner the kids were excused to watch TV, and the four adults continued to chat while sipping herb tea. "Don't sit too close to the set," cautioned Grandpa. "And don't watch if there's nothing worth watching." The kids were out of hearing, but Grandpa called after them with the same jokes repeated each time he sees them: "A picture used to be worth a thousand words. Then came television." And, "The kid next door watches so many commercials on TV, he asked his parents for bad breath."

"So how's your natural diet?" asked Grandpa, more seriously. "Mine stinks. I don't know why you want to torture yourselves. You're both young and healthy."

"Dad, we're enjoying our life-style changes, and so are the kids. We think our meals are terrific, and we've never felt better. But we don't call it a 'natural' diet. The word natural can mean anything or nothing. Would you like to hear what's in 'natural' chocolate ice cream?"

"No, but I'd like some."

Jane told him anyway.

" 'Natural' chocolate ice cream usually contains milk solids, liquid sugar, corn syrup (which is also sugar), cocoa (which has sugar in it), flavor (which means it's not real), carob bean gum, guar gum, carrageenan, karaya gum, mono- and diglycerides, and annato color."

"Sounds good to me!"

"We're trying to teach the kids that 'naturalness' exists in the food promoter's mind. 'Natural' potato chips could be made from potatoes soaked in lye, skin removed, high fat content added, depleted protein values. That's natural? The word has been oversimplified, draining it of any meaning. Yet it conjures up an image of nutritional quality. You can't reduce 'natural' to measurable numbers.[138] We don't want the kids to be influenced by the advertisements on TV. Here, Pop, I brought something for you to read."

The paper Jim handed his father-in-law contained a few abstracts written by Donald R. Davis, Ph.D., of the Clayton Foundation Biochemical Institute, in Austin, Texas:

DISMEMBERED FOOD

Americans derive a majority of their calories from dismembered foods which have lost all or most of the nutrients in whole foods. Dismembered foods are purified □sugars□, □separated fats□, □alcohol□, and □milled□ grains.

If pigs or cows were fed the typical American diet, without added vitamins and other supplements, the entire livestock industry could be wiped out.

Human beings must receive from their external environment about forty-five or more different substances which they cannot make internally; these substances are called ☆nutrients☆. These nutrients are also required in the makeup and functioning of the cells and tissues of plants and animals. We can be nourished when we eat the cells and tissues of plants and animals, and this is essentially how humans and all other creatures on earth have always received the nutrients they must have.

Substitutes for purified sugars, separated fats, and conventional white flour are little better than what they replace. Over half the calories consumed in the United States come, in effect, from a large piece of cake.[139]

—Donald R. Davis, Ph.D.

At this point Grandma said, "The children tell me they are not drinking milk anymore. I hope you know what you're doing. Where will they get their ☆calcium☆?"

"Don't worry, Mom, they get plenty of calcium. ☆Eggs☆, chicken, raw ☆**green leafy vegetables**☆, millet, nuts, and seeds—all these foods have calcium. And don't they look terrific? No more runny noses, no more colds."

"My grandchildren always look terrific. They have plenty of time to worry about diet. It seems impractical to make such changes. It's like turning them into patients."

"We are presenting the facts, and allowing them to make their decisions, within the limits that we set. Accepting and understanding good food here and now is the best gift we can give them. Ultimately, what it means for them is long life after youth."

Grandpa changed the subject. "I'm very confused about fats. Hard, soft, unsaturated, essential. Can you explain them to me?"

"Sure. You know, Pop, there's a lot of confusion even among nutritionists about healthful and unhealthful fats. For starters, an essential nutrient is anything that your body requires in its daily biochemical activity which it is unable to make by its own chemical processes. Your body can make all the parts of the fat molecules except for polyunsaturated fatty acids, called PUFAs.

"PUFAs are found in naturally occurring ☆vegetable☆ and ☆fish☆ oils, and in human milk. All you need is about a teaspoonful a day, but believe it or not, it's hard to find good, unprocessed oil.

"PUFAs are very chemically reactive. Because they are so reactive, they are affected by improper storage. They become rancid very easily. Early ▢rancidity of fat▢ is not detectable by smell or taste, but it does affect the usefulness of these PUFAs in the body. When PUFAs are rancid, it is because they are peroxidized, and this is the result of reacting with oxygen. Nature very wisely 'packages' these highly reactive substances with ☆**vitamin E**☆, which prevents peroxidation and, therefore, rancidity.

"Unfortunately, processing of oils removes most of the protective vitamin E. When you get your PUFAs from processed oils, like ▢**salad dressing**▢, it's a good idea to take vitamin E too—at least 100 units a day. Otherwise the healthful PUFAs in your body can be peroxidized and become toxic. If you are getting your PUFAs from whole foods, like fresh nuts and seeds (purchased in the shell), and avocados, the vitamin E is right there where it belongs, ready to do its police work.

"But it's not all that simple. Fat molecules are large and complex, and they have a specific configuration in space—a physical form. When we look at a glove, we can recognize that it was designed to fit a hand, but we also know that there are right hand and left hand gloves, and that one doesn't fit the other. They are mirror images, alike but not identical because they are reversed. Chemical molecular structures are also capable of having mirror image forms. Your body can use only the so-called *cis* form of fatty acids. That's the one that fits into your body machinery. In fact, it fits like a glove! But here's the rub: when fats are processed, we convert some of the cis fatty acids into *trans* configurations. And these trans fatty acids do not fit into the body machinery. Now you're trying to put the righthanded glove on the left hand, and this gums up the works.

"*All* ▫**processed**▫ fats have this unhealthful form of fatty acid. There is probably no healthful margarine available in the United States. Most, if not all, cooking oils and fats contain excessive quantities of trans fatty acids. So it's not only the question of saturated and unsaturated that must be considered, but also the processing, which produces the wrong fatty acid configuration. Ordinary saturated fat, such as that found in beef or chicken, is more healthful than the trans unsaturated fatty acids found in corn oil margarine.

"So, when you shop, avoid any package that says it contains hydrogenated vegetable oil, saturated vegetable oil, or hardened vegetable oil. Even partially hydrogenated is no good. As Carlton Fredericks says, 'Partially hydrogenated is like being a little bit pregnant.' There is no such thing as a solid polyunsaturated fat at room temperature. If you see something that is supposed to be high in PUFAs and it's solid, you know you're being ripped off. PUFAs are liquid at room temperature. Again, most 'pure' vegetable oil preparations are so highly processed, they contain the trans PUFAs, even though they aren't hardened. In general, the beautiful clear oils are too purified for good health, and butter is more healthful than margarine.

"One of the most important factors triggering ▫**rancidity in fat**▫ is exposure to excessive heat. PUFA-rich oils may be used for cooking, but only at low heat and for short cooking times. These oils, once opened, should be kept refrigerated, and used promptly. If not used in four months, they should be discarded and replaced. Typical oils high in PUFAs include safflower, sunflower, and sesame.

"Wait, don't go away. There's more. Let's say you've taken your PUFAs, and they're not rancid. Now your body has to convert the oil into a usable form. If you don't have enough ☆**vitamin C**☆, or you are deficient in B_6, or if you are □overweight□, have diabetes, or are a senior citizen, chances are you'll have difficulty making this conversion. Too many trans fatty acids in the diet also become an obstacle.

"The oils we've been talking about are called Omega-6 oils. There's another type of fatty acid called Omega-3. Omega-3 is found in fish-liver oils and linseed oil. Since linseed oil also contains Omega-6 PUFAs, it is highly recommended as a dietary supplement. However, it is not very tasty, and can also become rancid easily. Cod-liver oil is an excellent Omega-3 oil. Another good source is any ☆**fish**☆ from northern waters.[140] Eat salmon, halibut, striped bass, cod—and *eat the skin.* That's where the oils are concentrated."

Grandpa asked, "Would you run those omegas by me once more?"

"Sure. I'll explain it another way. All cell membranes are composed of PUFAs. Fish adapt to cold water by producing PUFAs which remain fluid at lower temperatures. They have to remain liquid to retain permeability, so that nutrients can penetrate the cell for energy and growth. Fish that live in warm waters do not need low temperature PUFAs because the more saturated fats will still be fluid at a warmer temperature. Butter, for example, a more saturated fat, will melt at room temperature, but harden in the refrigerator. If the fat in the cell membranes of the cold water fish were like butter, it would not be liquid enough for efficient cell function. Omega 3 describes the structure of the lower temperature PUFA, while Omega 6 indicates the fatty acid of the warm water fish. And that's 'oil' I know!"

Grandma and Grandpa both spoke at once.

"You're so smart. It's clear now."

"What do we do for □salad dressings□?"

"Jane can give you salad dressing recipes that use foods containing natural oils, like avocados and sunflower seeds. ☆**Yogurt**☆ is a good base for salad dressings too."

The children joined the adults, and Grandpa went into his act again. "Kids, you've got to help your old grandpa:

> No matter what my condition,
> Listen to me, please.
> For me the best physician
> Is apple pie and cheese.[141]

"Let's go get ten flavors of ice cream."

Much to Grandpa's surprise, the children said, "We're too good for that. Let's finish the Chinese leftovers."

MEG AND KEITH AND LE CHEZ CRÉCY

Fancy But Famished

Meg and Keith were in a dimly lit restaurant. The beautiful linen cloth was graced with freshly cut exotic hothouse flowers, artfully arranged. The champagne cooler looked all the more sophisticated for having Dom Pérignon in its care. The menu left much to be desired.

Mimi Sheraton, former restaurant reviewer for *The New York Times*, described the kitchen of a very busy and very fancy French restaurant. "I was surprised," she wrote, "to see a young chef sitting in a chair with his feet up on a table, reading a magazine. The only equipment in view was a large freezer and a microwave oven."

By the time they were seated, Meg knew too much about Keith. Her instinct had been to refuse his invitation, and she found herself wondering why she had accepted. Meg was sure that when he looked straight at her it was only to adjust his hair in the reflection of her glasses.

THE APPETIZER:
Crécy Glacé for Meg; *Jambon à la Crème* for Keith

Keith was confused when Meg asked the waiter if she could have a ☆**vegetable**☆ selection as an appetizer. "I can't imagine such a strong vegetable preference."

"French appetizers are too rich," explained Meg. Actually, she selected a vegetable because it appeared to be the least "fractured" of the items listed. Meg did not feel that this was the time or place to expound on her food attitudes. Nor did she want to sound like the reformers who believe in life, liberty, and the pursuit of *other* people's happiness.

Crécy Glacé

The carrots looked exquisite. They were tiny baby carrots, seasoned with salt, MSG, and lemon juice, and then sautéed in margarine. □**Sugar**□ and honey were added to produce a golden glaze.

Meg refrained from sharing with Keith:

• Her disdain for foods cooked with salt, MSG, margarine, sugar, and honey.

- Her discovery that adding grated carrots to her daily salad had an amazingly beneficial effect on ameliorating constipation.
- Her choice of carrots over other vegetables because of her nutritionist's explanations of the association of good skin health and ☆**vitamin A**☆. Carrots contain provitamin A, (which her body should convert to vitamin A), and even ☆**vitamins B, C, and E**☆, plus ☆**trace elements**☆: iron, magnesium, calcium, and phosphorus.

Meg may not have been able to get a word in anyway. Keith's favorite topic was Keith. At the moment, he was explaining his ▢**nicotine**▢ addiction, and trying to be humorous about it. "When people give up smoking, they substitute something for it: irritability. I once gave up cigarettes and started chewing toothpicks, but I developed Dutch elm disease. And I'm glad I don't have to explain to Martians why I set fire to dozens of little pieces of paper, and then put them in my mouth. Ha! Ha!"

Jambon à la Crême

What a fancy name for ham with cream sauce! The ingredients include shallots, white wine vinegar, margarine, flour, beef stock, dry white wine, salt, pepper, heavy cream, and breadcrumbs.

When Keith offered Meg a taste, she refused. She had to respond to his persistence with some degree of honesty. "I'm allergic to anything with milk." That was as close to the truth as she could get. She did not add that she was also sensitive to toxic ideas, such as the politics involved in allowing the use of nitrites in that ham.

THE SALAD:
Salade des Endives et des Oranges for Meg; *Tomates Farcies* for Keith

Salade des Endives et des Oranges

This was not Meg's day. (It was certainly not her restaurant.) She anticipated that at least the *salade* would provide offerings of whole food. Endive and orange salad was the least offensive salad on the menu.

When people begin to eat real food, unmasked, without ▢**additives**▢, they discover that they develop a heightened sensitivity to taste. Meg would not have noticed subtle rancidity six months ago. Now corruptions such as too many trans-fat molecules in a salad dressing announce themselves with trumpet blasts. Before all these indignities were bestowed on food, people depended on their senses to determine food quality. Artificial colors and flavors often destroy this ability.

The endive was drowning in □rancid vinaigrette□, seasoned with □sugar□. Meg had forgotten to say to the waiter, "Dressing on the side, please." But the greatest vulgarity was the lack of orange in "Salade des Endives et des Oranges." For Meg, this caption conjured up an image of crisp sheets of endive, embellished with fresh orange slices. Grated orange rind was the reality.

An article in *The New York Times* assessed the effects of chemically treated food, oranges in particular:

A fresh Florida orange is one example of how some foods are currently treated: after being harvested, it is washed with detergent to remove pesticides, mold, and dirt. A fungicide is sprayed on to retard rotting. Then, to satisfy consumer preference for orange-colored oranges, the naturally greenish Florida fruit may be dyed by using ethylene gas and a red coloring agent that some studies have linked to bladder cancer in laboratory animals (the growers dispute the relevance of the findings). As a final sprucing, and to prevent excessive moisture loss, a petroleum-based wax or a shellac is applied and the fruit is sometimes buffed.

. . . The FDA permits the dye citrus red No. 2 to be used on oranges, but only in tiny amounts—two parts per million by weight. Consumer groups contend that the dye should be prohibited because it is superfluous and, possibly, a carcinogen in humans.

In 1977 the Public Health Research Group, a Ralph Nader organization, petitioned the agency to ban this and other food dyes. The petition cited a number of international studies, including one sponsored by the World Health Organization, that indicated that citrus red dye No. 2 is a carcinogen in animals, according to Dr. Sidney M. Wolfe, director of the research group. . . . After a review of the scientific studies, the FDA reaffirmed its limited approval of the dye in 1979.

Growers comply for the most part with the Federal and State labeling laws by listing the waxes, chemicals, and colors used on fruit and vegetables, but retailers generally fail to display the cases bearing the labels or to post appropriate notices.

Waxes have not been subjected to rigorous laboratory and clinical testing of additives. The waxes on food are similar to those used to shine and seal floors and polish automobiles. Derived from petroleum and natural sources, they often contain some combination of paraffin, shellac, canauba, polyethylene, and synthetic resins. The wax, which cannot be washed off because it has a high melting temperature, is also used as a vehicle for applying a wide variety of bactericides, fungicides, growth regulators, and dyes. The safety of ingesting shellac is still under review. Since it is used to coat jelly beans, President Reagan's favorite candy, the President is the No. 1 guinea pig. Prominent among colored produce are "new" or "red" potatoes and sweet potatoes. It is illegal, however, for a yellow sweet potato to be dyed red because the FDA considers that a deceptive practice. The agency has the authority to seize such deceptive products and impose a fine, but has not done so in recent years.[142]

Meg may not have eaten the orange anyway. Citrus fruit was on her "no" list. Her nutritionist had explained that the farther you live from California and Florida, where the oranges grow, the more likely you are to be sensitive to them.

Meg's salad had one redeeming feature: it was wreathed with watercress. Growing as it does in running water, watercress is naturally rich in ☆vitamins☆ and ☆minerals☆ and is unaffected by soil erosion. The high sulphur content gives it a pungent flavor which stimulates the appetite and helps pick up bland foods so that condiments such as salt and pepper are unnecessary. (Judging from the salt in the vinaigrette, this bit of information is unknown to the chef at Le Chez Crécy.)

Tomates Farcies

Tomatoes stuffed with vegetables and rice. But why did they smother the filling with so much mayonnaise? What are they trying to cover up?

Meg could have shared this bit of tomato trivia:

Tomatoes used to be a garden ornament. And it's not a vegetable, but a fruit. It's even listed as a berry. When the tomato first arrived in America, it was considered beautiful, but poisonous. Tomatoes are an important source of ☆vitamin C☆ and provide a generous amount of provitamin A.

Placing tomatoes on the window sill to ripen is not a good idea. Too much sunlight prevents development of normal or even color. Green tomatoes will ripen well if kept in a dry place, light or dark, at a temperature of 55 to 70 degrees. Once they're ripe, they should be refrigerated and kept dry.

Meg chose not to discuss tomatoes because she was sure the only tomato that would hold Keith's interest would be one with 36–24–36 measurements.

THE ENTREE:
Bar Farci aux Huitres et Aubergine for Meg; *Foie de Veau Smitane* for Keith

Bar Farci aux Huitres et Aubergine

Baked bass with oyster stuffing and eggplant was the only main dish without a milk-based sauce and/or excessive wheat garnishings. The stuffing did contain breadcrumbs, but a minimal amount, according to the waiter. Yogurt, not cream, was the enrichment here.

The waiter praised the filets de soles, but Meg rejected his suggestion. Meg has a difficult time eating either flounder or sole ever since a fisherman told her that these flat, bottom-dwelling fish are scavengers, and too close to shore for comfort. Her choice is confirmed with her new knowledge of the importance of Omega-3 essential fatty acids, found in deep ocean ☆**fish**☆ of northern waters.

The advantages of Omega-3 essential fatty acids came to light in studies of the traditional Eskimo diet, which is very high in protein, fat, cholesterol, and retinol (☆**vitamin A**☆), and low in fiber and tocopherols (vitamin E). The traditional Eskimo, however, has low blood cholesterol and an absence of noninfective Western diseases (such as cancer, arthritis, diabetes, and so on).[143,144] The fat of the Arctic marine animals is the most unsaturated found among animals, being particularly rich in the Omega-3 class of oils.[145] There is no doubt that fatty fish can greatly lower blood triglycerides, lower the bad guy fractions of cholesterol (LDL and VLDL—low density lipoproteins and very low density lipoproteins), and raise the good guy fractions (HDL—high density lipoproteins), as well as decrease platelet aggregation. (Dr. Bob Smith's colleagues should be swallowing herring and mackerel rather than aspirin!)

The mystery is that fish oils contain little vitamin E. This is no problem when fresh fish is consumed, but the oils do get rancid easily when extracted from the fish.[146] In general, Meg enjoys anything that lives in the sea and finds its way to the table.

Although the stuffing was a bit salty for her reeducated taste buds, she enjoyed the bass.

Foie de Veau Smitane

It was clear that Keith believed that all he had to do was run, run, run, and he could cheat, cheat, cheat. Meg was surprised that Keith ordered anything as healthful as liver.

The *Foie de Veau Smitane* was an extravaganza of adornments and preparation, especially compared to the *bonne bouche* that Meg prepares in fifteen minutes, and which she calls "Liver Slivers." The fancy French version includes a coating of flour, involved cuisine artistry, and a sour cream dressing comprised of twelve ingredients.

Although liver has long been esteemed a health food of value, many people hesitate to eat it. Here's the controversy:

- Liver antagonists claim that because the liver is a detoxifying organ, toxins settle in its tissue. Don't eat it.
- Liver proponents claim that since the liver is a detoxifying organ, it gets rid of toxins. Eat it. Besides, toxins settle in fat throughout the body. If the toxins are concentrated in the liver, the liver is not doing its job.

The reason it's at issue at all is that we consume very little organ meat. Organ meats are the most nutritious of all meats, and liver is queen of the organ meats. Because of its vital role in digestion, it is a depot of all vitamins and minerals taken into the body. (Native American tribes believed the human liver to be the repository of manly virtues, such as courage.[147])

A quick comparison of a few of the nutrients in liver and in hamburger graphically demonstrates the superiority of liver:

	Hamburger (4oz)	*Liver* (4oz)
Iron	2.8 mgs	7.8 mgs
Vitamin A	none	53,500 units
Vitamin C	none	31 mgs

DESSERT:
Poires Belle Hélène à la Caroube For Meg; *Tarte des Demoiselles Tatin* for Keith

Poires Belle Hélène à la Caroube

Meg said, "None, thanks," when the waiter asked for dessert choices. The gentleman looked as though he was hurt to the quick.

He then smiled graciously, and said, "Let me charm you." And he did, as he reeled off descriptions of end-of-meal temptations.

"Here's where I blow it," thought Meg. Keith said, "You have such a superb figure. Have dessert; it'll never show. Just run a little more tomorrow. That's what I do."

It would have been pointless to explain. The poached pears with carob sauce surprised Meg. They were not sweet, and were spruced up with nuts.

Tarte des Demoiselles Tatin

Keith said he always selected a dessert with fruit, because fruit was *natural.* Such innocence! Apple upside-down tart is made with □sugar□, and more sugar, and more sugar. The final step is caramelizing the top with *more* sugar. Natural?

Not one action of sugar can be considered beneficial. Far too many actions of sugar are disastrous. To cite but a few:

- A study reported in *Metabolism* demonstrated that feeding sucrose to animals who are prone to hypertension raises blood pressure.[148]
- Maintaining test animals on a high sugar diet during gestation and lactation influences the activity levels of their offspring.[149]
- Beet sugar sensitivity has been reported in medical books.[150] It is not uncommon to have sugar allergies.
- High sugar intake contributes to hypoglycemia and diabetes.[151] It has been said that Mark Twain advised that "the secret to success in life is to eat what you like and let the food fight it out inside." Dr. Carl Pfeiffer, of the Princeton Brain Bio Center, comments that "the food is indeed 'fighting it out inside' and in too many cases wholly defeating the glucose regulatory mechanisms."[152]
- The factors involved in the increase in coronary heart disease are complex, but the increased consumption of refined carbohydrate in the form of sugar is a major contributor.[153]

Omnipresent Salt

A substance used liberally in almost every preparation was salt. We have learned a great deal about salt from no-salt cultures. One such culture is that of the Yanomama Indians of South America. Dr. William Oliver has studied the Yanomama Indians, and Meg read a fascinating article on the results:

NO-SALT CULTURES:
A CONSIDERATION IN DIETARY GUIDELINES IN OUR MODERN SOCIETIES

A possible important consideration for the role of salt in nutrition is a knowledge of the information available from studies of those societies who have had no access to salt in its crystalline form and who seem to have sustained no adverse affect from its absence.

My colleagues and I observed that salt was absent in the culture of the Yanomama Indians of South America. Subsequently, in the course of physical examinations to assess the general health of these isolated, unacculturated people, we further observed that blood pressure did not increase with age as occurs in industrialized societies. It was then decided to study their salt balance and the bodily adjustments permitting health and survival despite an absence of salt.

It is known in man and in comparative animals [descending even to *low* animals] that a hormonal system exists to promote the retention of salt by the kidneys, as well as the sweat glands and the gastrointestinal tract in higher animals.

The impressively low blood pressure observed in the Yanomama cannot be attributed to a lack of stressful environment. Within the village the men believe they must create a consistent macho image among their peers; between villages there are frequent raids to avenge perceived or valid insults and to secure brides. Life for the Yanomama is not a serene existence in a jungle paradise, but rather a daily struggle to gain and maintain respect from one's fellow tribesmen and for simple survival.

To place these observations in appropriate perspective, it should be understood that the Yanomama are not unique in respect to absence of salt in the diet. Other groups who were without salt at the time of initial contact include an aboriginal ethnic group in the Szechwan Province of Western China, the Masai of Africa, certain Indians of North America, the Melanesians of the interior of New Guinea, the Polynesian inhabitants of the Pukapuka atoll in the South Pacific, and the Tasaday of the Philippines.[154]

To turn to a different facet in respect to dietary salt, it is well documented that individuals in our society possess the physiological adaptations to maintain health when restricted to salt intake only slightly exceeding that of the unacculturated Yanomama Indian. In the mid-1940s, drugs promoting salt excretion were not available and severe dietary restriction of salt intake was successfully tested for the treatment of malignant, life-threatening high blood pressure. This was the era of the medically famed Kempner rice-fruit-sugar diet. Of historic interest is the fact that the first formal proposal that reduction of salt intake potentially could ameliorate high blood pressure was made early in this century.[155]

In as yet unpublished studies we found that the ability of Yanomama Indian infants to conserve salt matched that of their parents. We could deduce no reason from either our observations or from our physical examinations of infants, children, and adults to suggest that the daily quantity of salt required for realization of full growth potential could not be met by that amount naturally present in food, including breast milk.

Taken in toto, these observations have significant implications for the optimal quantity of salt in the diet. The Report of the Senate Select Committee on Nutrition and Human Needs suggested a drastic reduction in salt intake from present levels.[156]

Existence of an appetite for salt in man and lower animals is well known. All of us are familiar with individuals who routinely salt their food prior to even the first taste, to the dismay of a gourmet hostess or fastidious chef. In studies of infants, it has been shown that those less than six months of age are quite indifferent to various concentrations of salt in solution. However, by two years of age, and perhaps earlier, children of our society will preferentially choose salted foods over those containing no added salt.[157] Obviously, this preference continues throughout life, as we well know.

Recommendations for dietary salt cannot be based on quantities that provide a "good taste" since the innate salt appetite will induce use of amounts far in excess of need. The salt content naturally present in a well-balanced diet will provide a sufficient quantity of that mineral for healthy individuals.[158]

—William Oliver, M.D.

It's of interest to note that the FDA allows the sodium content of products to vary as much as 120 percent from the value on the label because the sodium content of water used in manufacturing varies from city to city. Sodium content also varies in different samples of a given commodity.[159]

Goodnight (and Goodbye) Keith

The final insult of this incredibly expensive dinner was the serving of chocolate candies with the bill. "How delightful," said Keith. "How ridiculous," thought Meg. Her first refusal of the candies was not followed by further proddings. (Keith probably wanted all the chocolate for himself.)

Had Meg eaten the chocolate, she would have developed a head-ache. Had she drunk the wine, her migraine would have been something to write home about.

Many drinkers of red wine are affected by migraine type head-aches, and don't realize the cause. Some red wines contain high amounts of histamine.[160,161] Doctors in California wine country report that white wine may also precipitate migraine. They state that it is more common in inexpensive jug wine and in bottled wine that has been open some days before drinking. A person will note that when a bottle of wine is opened and partly consumed, there are no symptoms. But when the wine is later removed from the refrigerator and finished, a nasty and lasting headache may ensue. Chablis and mixed white wines more often cause the symptoms than do the "better" white wines.

As for chocolate, the dark is more apt to create a headache than is light chocolate. Some people experience the problem only when chocolate and □coffee□ are consumed simultaneously. Sometimes an upset stomach will accompany the headache. It was noted that head-ache does not occur, or will occur much less frequently, if the food-stuff is consumed in the morning, but the symptoms will invariably appear if taken before sleep.[162]

Keith talked on: "I tried health foods once, but it was so embar-rassing, getting drunk on eggnog. What can you say to people—you're under the influence of cinnamon?"

Observing Keith on the track, Meg assumed he had a fervent de-votion to physical well-being. Having spent the evening with him, she realized that running was his only expression of a healthful life-style. His view of what is healthful is very narrow. Diet, other forms of ex-ercise, social habits, recreation, and work patterns, which are very vi-tal aspects of living, were considered of lesser importance.

★   ★   ★

Gluttony is not a secret vice.

—Orson Welles

The unfortunate thing about this world is that good habits are so much easier to give up than bad ones.

—Somerset Maugham

I would sooner surrender my rights than my habits.

—Everyperson

CHAPTER 5

═══════════════════════════════════════

═══════════════════════════════════════

The Stress Effect

═══════════════════════════════════════

═══════════════════════════════════════

Middle age is when you want to see how long your car will last and not how fast it will go; when you still believe you'll feel better in the morning; when your phone rings at home on a Saturday night and you hope it isn't for you; and when you are told to slow down by a doctor instead of a policeman.

WISDOM FROM MA SMITH

═══════════════════════════════════════

Stress And Today's Food

When Bob was a child, his mother scolded him when he cried at the dinner table. The reprimand, explained his Mom, had nothing to do with her annoyance at his behavior. "You see," she would say, "when you shed tears while eating, food turns to poison."

It was many years later that Bob learned that digestion does indeed start in one's head. *There is an intimate relationship between emotional stress and gastrointestinal malabsorption.*

It is no surprise to Bob that in today's world there are more allergies, an increase in hypoglycemia (low blood sugar), diabetes, and an overwhelming profusion of other degenerative diseases such as lupus (a serious inflammatory disease of the skin or connective tissue that could be fatal), arthritis, cancer, heart disease, and presenile dementia (a condition resembling senility, but occurring in early or middle life).

Bob devours every article that details just how the impoverished

158

quality of our food (plus the commercial □processing□ it undergoes) is responsible for nutrient depletion. He understands how, when confronted with pressures, this fault in the foodways of our country places his patients (and his own family) at a higher risk of disease. Combining the intake of "plastic" foods with emotional stress creates a negative effect, one that is geometrically cumulative. Foods of the late twentieth century are poor sources of nutrients compared with more natural foods. Another of Bob's fact sheets attempts to convey this concept to his patients (part of which has been extrapolated from a presentation by Serafina Corsello, M.D., medical director of the renowned Stress Center in Huntington, L.I., N.Y.[1]):

UNPLEASANT IMAGES AND WHAT YOUR BRAIN DOES WITH THEM

Stress begins its destructive action at the level of the midbrain. A disagreement with either your boss or a client may be an upsetting event. The image of the altercation travels from your cortex (the outer layer of gray matter in your brain which receives sensory stimuli) to your brain's deeper structures. One of the most important of these deep structures is the hypothalamus, which works like a dispatching station of a telecommunications center. Once it receives the message of an uncomfortable or dangerous situation, it sends stimulating impulses to its entire territory. One of the reactions which then ensues is the production of adrenalin.[2] How many times have you heard and used the expression, "My adrenalin was flowing," a statement denoting excitation. But that's just the tip of the iceberg. *The hypothalamus has been considered as the possible primary site triggering the onset of aging at the level of the whole organism.*[3]

The might of your hypothalamus puts the seventeenth-century British Empire to shame. Your hypothalamus is in command of activating, empowering, and integrating your autonomic mechanisms (those which are self-controlled and which function without conscious effort). These include endocrine activities (those responsible for hormonal secretions), and many other functions such as fluid regulation, body temperature control, sleep patterns, and even food intake.[4]

The hypothalamus is top kingpin of your brain's relay setup. And it alerts *all of you* to unpleasant or threatening situations. That's the stress effect. All of you reacts, and does so with the speed of an electronic messenger.

Of special concern are the functions that occur automatically in the large organs of your body—contractions of your heart, the movement of your gut, *the secretion of digestive enzymes,* the process of perspiring, to name but a few. All of this happens without your awareness, but in response to events that you are experiencing. Your reactions to any episode may be pleasing or displeasing, and your body responds accordingly.

This base of operations controlling your body without your conscious dictate is divided into two networks called sympathetic and parasympathetic autonomic nervous systems. An important distinction between these two branches is that the sympathetic is stimulated at times of stress; the parasympathetic regulates, among many other physiological processes, restorative or peaceful functions, including the secretion of gastrointestinal enzymes.

Your interpretation of circumstances signals the command for either (but not both) of these systems to prevail. For example, if you are sitting quietly at home reading a delightful novel with a beautiful rendition of Beethoven's Ninth Symphony in the background, your parasympathetic system is operating. If lightning suddenly strikes a tree outside your window, your sympathetic system takes over. You feel the stress effect immediately.

A serious problem develops when you are repeatedly faced with stressors. Lightning doesn't strike twice, but your kids might. Your teenager may be causing you grief on a daily basis, or you may be constantly stirring the embers of your sympathetic system because your mother-in-law is intruding morning, noon, and night. These events cause the same activation of your stress mechanisms as that bolt of lightning.

When distressing events occur often enough, you find yourself in a constant state of high arousal, which is independent of the stimulus. In other words, the sympathetic system becomes the master even at times when you should be relaxed. People with such a condition will demonstrate elevated muscle tension and body movement. You've all seen the ill-at-ease child twirling hair; the teenager repeatedly tapping a foot; the adult poking with a pencil. These people often lose the ability to shift into the parasympathetic, or calm mode of behavior, even when they should be free of tension.

You can see what a vicious cycle this becomes: the muscle tension results in propagating more stimuli for the sympathetic system. All this "over-firing" is at the expense of the central nervous system, and it is often referred to as the burn-out syndrome. The consequences can even modify brain function.[5]

Not all stress, however, is caused by the "driven" lifestyle. A person who feels unaccomplished and unfulfilled in a lack-luster world also experiences stress.

—Bob Smith, M.D.

Bob asks his patients to question him after reading this information. It is his hope that understanding the concepts outlined will facilitate change.

Another concern is the continuously multiplying use of tranquilizers. It appears that the yearly rate of increase will lead to the total tranquilization of America by the turn of the century.[6] Perhaps the trend will reverse because of awareness created through scientific publications and the lay press, which suggest dramatic consequences and hazards of tranquilizer use.[7,8,9,10] Maybe.

BEN'S STRESS PHILOSOPHY

An Inheritance From Caveperson

It all goes back to the caveperson, says Ben. There is no doubt that human beings have made tremendous strides from the time the latest Christian Dior was a homemade animal skin, and a club, instead of the hydrogen bomb, was the weapon of mass destruction. The progression of change from cave dwelling to Lindbergh's transatlantic crossing spanned millions of years. Ben points out that the incredible technological advances of the last fifty years make *all* the change known to humankind up to that time a mere fribble—a storm in a teacup. The pace of life has now acquired a rhythm that has become more frantic than our ability to cope with such changes, or even to comprehend many of them.

Ben agrees with philosophers who refer to the twentieth century as the Age of Uncertainty, the Age of Anxiety, the Age of Rapid Change, and even Future Shock—the writers who explain that our perception of external events has assumed a more threatening quality. The hypothalamus is sending messages of "war" to internal organs with increasing frequency. However, our physiology is still the physiology of caveperson. We have not evolved with the kind of efficiency that allows differentiation between a mugger going after us with a knife, or symbolic threatening situations such as displeasure after an argument with a spouse, anxiety experienced in a traffic jam, or the trauma of too few hours in the day to complete all goals. And we go through the stress effect again and again and again. And again.

Phobias and fears are widespread and divergent. Ben enjoys telling the story of an event that occurred in his family years back. Driving over bridges made his wife cower. His daughter envisions hell as a place full of tunnels. Vacationing together, Ben's family set out from New York, heading for the shores of New Jersey. There are two ways to get across the Hudson River: bridge and tunnel. Ben cooperated, and leaving the bridge loather behind, drove his daughter over the river; then he went back to get his wife and drove her through the tunnel. Not everyone has such an understanding chauffeur. For those who don't, the end product is □**stress**□.

Ben recognizes that the physiology of caveperson was geared to very basic functions aimed primarily at survival. Gathering of food, reproduction, and protection of the herd were prime objectives. When caveperson went out to search for food, supplies were often totally diminished. It is unlikely that prehistoric man of the house (cave?) commenced his quest with a meal in his stomach.

As it happens, the first thing to be disrupted when under stress is the ability to digest food and consequently extract nutrients (vitamins and minerals) from this food. This is due to the fact that the stimulus perceived as threatening through that figure of authority in the brain, the hypothalamus, has sent stress messages to internal organs. Since these organs are not essential for *immediate* survival, blood is diverted from them to the big muscles of arms and legs—so important in the "fight or flight" mechanism. Ben knows that we need a lot of blood in our vessels to run, or to fight. As the message races through the body, organs squeeze out blood. Spleen (which is the greatest reservoir of blood), liver, and kidneys all get into the act. The heart is also asked to work faster and stronger in order to pump more blood into muscles. The body is prepared for action, *and all digestive functions cease.* (This explains the diarrhea that some people experience following a stressful event. When the system returns to normal, the body has to deal with undigested food.)

Ben read a fascinating article which explained that digestion is not necessary for primary survival, but when stress occurs as frequently as it does in our society, long-range survival is ultimately undermined by the onset of destructive degenerative disease. The reason? Mainly because we are not absorbing nutrients from our food. Criticism or being late for an appointment creates the same stress effect as experienced by caveperson confronting a wild animal, but now the body has to deal with digestion at the same time.

Ben has concluded that his pace, and that of his peers, is more like caveperson's. As for the younger generations, they are double-parked most of the time.

GRANDMA IS RIGHT AGAIN

TV News and Dinner

In his quest for scientific information about diets for exercisers, Mike discovered a fascinating □stress□/digestion connection. There is a constant delicate balance between the sympathetic and parasympathetic systems—the two networks controlled by the hypothalamus. The sympathetic system triggers production of adrenalin. Again, everyone knows that adrenalin means excitation. The parasympathetic system is responsible for production of acetylcholine, which produces the relaxation response. When imbalances exist between these two chemicals, you are unable to secrete the gastrointestinal juices necessary for proper digestion. It has even been proposed that the terms sympathetic and parasympathetic be replaced by adrenergic (meaning stimulated, activated, or transmitted by adrenalin) and cholinergic (meaning stimulated, activated, or transmitted by choline).[11]

Although our ancestors were certainly not cognizant of these fine physiological patterns, their empirical observations and common sense suggested practices that helped them survive with greater ease. "How true," thought Mike. At times of distress, his Grandma discouraged heavy meals rich in foods that required many enzymes for digestion. Grandma told Mike that he should never eat a greasy hamburger on his way to an important business meeting at which he was scheduled to present a report. Or if his boss happened to say to him as he was leaving for his lunch break, "See me after lunch—we have to talk," he should eat a salad for lunch that day. Until recently, Mike had only smiled at Grandma's admonitions.

Mike has concluded that one of the most distressing intrusions on his physiological balance occurs when he is having dinner while watching the news. Not that watching the eleven o'clock news is a better choice. If he views the news at six, his digestion is affected. If he views the news at the late hour, he winds up exercising: tossing and turning in bed. And all because his hypothalamus is reading his emotions.

When the Lion Lies Down With the Lamb

When Mike's world is at peace, macronutrients—proteins, fats, and carbohydrates—are used to rebuild tissues and to provide energy. Very simply, this is how it works:

(1) Amino acids are broken down from the protein consumed, and are reassembled into human protein, as expressed or conditioned by Mike's genetic code. His body takes something else and converts it into Mike.

(2) Glucose, not to be confused with refined sugar, is the most immediate source of energy. The brain is its greatest utilizer. Physiologically speaking, glucose is the fastest and most economical source of energy. Mike can easily relate to this. He knows how he feels after he's eaten something sweet. The glucose not needed for energy at the moment is stored mostly as glycogen, or animal sugar. This is meant to be a reserve for times of famine.

(3) Fatty acids also enter into the burner for energy. If they are underutilized, they too are stored as reserves, put away as fatty deposits known as adipose tissue. These deposits are very hard to dispose of. (So it may have been the stress in his life that has kept the scale reading too high.)

Each individual cell is in essence a laboratory in which all of these events occur. But the stress response shuts down the digestive process responsible for these conversions. The proteins, fats, and carbohydrates of which food is comprised may simply not break down when the hypothalamus receives unpleasant images. If Mike is not in a relaxation posture when eating, he will not be able to properly extract:

1. amino acids from protein
2. glucose from carbohydrates
3. fatty acids and glycerol from fats

The same food that can nourish and nurture now becomes a burden. And a significant fact often overlooked is that the same stress that curtails the breaking down of food also puts the skids on nutrient supplements. *If you are not absorbing nutrients from food, the chances are you are not absorbing nutrients contained in a tablet or capsule.*

MIKE, MEG, AND THE STRESS SYMPOSIUM

Disruption Is Not Limited to Digestion

Mike's brother (the dentist) offered him two tickets to a medical symposium on stress. Mike invited Meg, and to his delight, she accepted.

The first lecturer quoted Hans Selye, renowned for his theories on stress, and his discussion on resistance to disease:

By *general resistance* I mean the ability to remain healthy—or at least alive—during intense stress caused nonspecifically by various agents . . .

Among newborn infants of foreign women employed in Germany as "guest workers" during an economic boom period, the malformation rate was unusually high, and this has been ascribed to the stressor effect of relocation into an unusual environment.

In guinea pigs and mice exposed to heat during certain stages of pregnancy, embryonic mortality and malformations—particularly brain damage—were often detectable. Various malformations of the brain have also been reported in the offspring of pregnant mice kept under extremely crowded conditions.

Aging itself—and particularly premature aging—is, in a sense, due to the constant, and eventually exhausting, stresses of life.[12]

The lecturer stated that Hans Selye's comments support the view that the disruption of physiological processes caused by stress may be the villain in many degenerative diseases as well as a cause of abnormalities.

The lecturer intrigued the audience when he said, "If the human brain were so simple that we could understand it, we would be so simple that we couldn't."[13] He then cited the results of a few studies which punctuate other disturbances incurred by stress:

- Endorphins are substances produced in your brain. They are self-made morphine. It is your built-in mechanism for easing pain. Endorphins are believed to have a profound effect on mood, which correlates with a sense of well-being.[14] In response to mild stress, the levels of endorphins in test animals fall significantly.[15] This is one reason why you feel more pain when you are under stress.

- Under certain conditions, your body releases its own opiates (again, pain-relieving substances). These secretions increase at times of stress, but they inhibit intestinal secretions necessary for digestion.[16] This is why you are more prone to digestive disorders when under stress.

- Collagen is a fibrous protein found in connective tissue, bone, and cartilage. There is a relationship between the production of this kind of protein in the arteries and the atherosclerotic process. Stress promotes the manufacture of collagen.[17] This is one connection between stress and heart disease.

- When under stress, you secrete hormones which reduce the efficacy of the white blood cells which are called T-cells, the body's soldier cells. T-cells are involved in defense. Artificial chemical stress has been produced by injecting an animal with the stress hormone.[18] This is why stress reduces your immunity to infection.
- Stress can increase the triglyceride fraction of blood fat by 50 percent.[19] (Triglycerides are the storage form of fat considered so important in the development of heart disease.) Here is another stress/heart disease connection.
- People viewing sexually arousing films with others present, medical students who have just taken an oral exam, and a group being interviewed for a job all proved to have something in common: a rise in free fatty acids in their blood. Free fatty acids are organic acids that combine with glycerin (a sugar) to form fat. Even mild emotional stress produces a rise in free fatty acids in your blood. The researchers conclude that chronic anxiety probably leads to chronic elevation of fatty acids in the blood.[20] This is why cholesterol levels go up when you are under stress.[21]
- When test animals are isolated, thereby placing them under stress, the muscular tissue of their hearts has very low magnesium levels.[22] This is one reason why loneliness actually causes physical impairment.
- When test animals are injected with the hormones secreted under stress, they are more likely to develop cancer.[23] This is why it has been theorized that people under stress are more likely to be cancer victims.
- The effect of academic stress on immunity was measured in dental students by checking their salivary secretions for immunoglobulin, the protein that has antibody activity. The immunoglobulin secretion rate was significantly lower in high-stress than low-stress periods for the whole group.[24]
- People undergoing a substantial number of life-change events show an increased incidence of allergic responses.[25]
- Experimental stress (stress initiated on test animals in the laboratory) is associated with an increase in the number and severity of dental caries.[26]
- The incidence of infectious mononucleosis among West Point cadets was highest among those in academic difficulty and whose parents had invested most in their success.[27]

There Is No Stress Disease

The keynote speaker startled the audience with his opening comment that there is no such thing as a stress disease. When the reactions of the audience simmered down, the speaker went on to say:

"If your stress mechanisms are well nourished, they will not break down." [And in fact, that's what *In Pursuit of Youth* is all about.] If your stress mechanisms are well nourished, you will have life after youth. Nor should it be forgotten that your perception of stress may be altered by judicious relaxation, resignation, and philosophy because emotional stress is your *personalized interpretation* of external events. Two drivers, each late for an appointment, each waiting for the traffic light to change, may have different reactions. One is chewing his fingernails, or digging them into the steering wheel. The other is calm and accepting. His attitude is: 'If it is not in my control, I will not let it get to me.' The traffic light is the stressor for only one of the drivers. Again, repeated acute stressors result in chronic stress symptoms.

"Hans Selye makes the statement that 'we could enormously lengthen the average human life-span by living in better harmony with natural laws.' "[28]

Following the lecture, Meg shared a humorous incident. "My sister and a girlfriend had not seen each other for a while. They met at a cocktail party. Each inquired about the other's children. My sister's friend said, 'Oh, I've had my hands full. Terrible problems!' My sister offered sympathy, but said, 'My kids are great.' When the distressed friend shared the details of her nonconforming children's disturbing exploits, my sister remained silent. My nieces were doing the same things, but my sister interpreted the new generation's activities as admirable." Their conversation typified some of the lecturers' points: stress is not so much what is happening, but how you react to what is happening.

Mike quoted one of the statements he had just heard: "And stress is what you anticipate will happen tomorrow—not only what actually happened yesterday."

SALLY ASSAYS TOM'S STRESS

The Stress Test

Sally began to wonder if Tom's stress was entirely negative. Time and again Tom said, "I thrive on stress." She was beginning to realize that exercise is physical stress that could have positive health value. Since the work of the hypothalamus isn't always palpable, is it possible to discern whether or not someone is a "stressed" person? Sally found a guide, adapted from *Inner Balance: The Power of Holistic Healing*, edited by Dr. Elliott Goldwag.

You may be under negative stress if you perceive yourself as:

1. generally irritable, hyperexcited, or depressed;
2. having a heart which you can hear pounding;
3. having dryness of the throat and mouth;
4. behaving impulsively, with aggression and emotional instability (emotion winning over logic);
5. experiencing overpowering urges to cry or to run and hide;
6. unable to concentrate, having flight of thoughts, and being generally disoriented;
7. accident prone;
8. having feelings of unreality, weakness, or dizziness;
9. feeling fatigued and going through the day without *joie de vivre*;
10. having "floating anxiety," afraid without cause;
11. emotionally tense, alert, and keyed up;
12. experiencing sexual difficulties, amenorrhea, impotence, premenstrual tension, or the "Casanova complex," nymphomania;
13. trembling, with nervous tics;
14. easily startled by small sounds;
15. laughing with a nervous high pitch;
16. stuttering, or having other speech difficulties, which are frequently stress-induced;
17. having bruxism, grinding of the teeth;
18. unable to sleep, a consequence of being keyed up;
19. having an increased tendency to move about or gesticulate without any apparent reason;
20. sweating excessively;
21. urinating frequently;
22. experiencing diarrhea, constipation, indigestion, queasiness in the stomach, even throwing up;

23. having no appetite, or an excessive one, showing itself in altera-
    tions of body weight—either excessive leanness or obesity;
24. experiencing pain in the neck or lower back;
25. having migraine headaches;
26. increasing smoking habits;
27. using additional prescribed medications, particularly tranquilizers
    or amphetamines;
28. addicted to alcohol or drugs;
29. experiencing nightmares;
30. experiencing neurotic behavior or even severe mental illness.[29]

Sally could not get Tom to sit down long enough to answer the questions. She didn't want to add to his stress by insisting. Nor could she answer the questions for him. Her perception of how he sees himself would be different from his self-impressions. When he revealed that the main reason why he consented to the plastic surgery was that he felt it would be better for his business image (those new executives were so young), she tried a new tack to encourage the exercise. She kept telling him how much younger it would make him look and feel.

A friend of Sally's who is a psychotherapist said, "I worry a lot. I worry about people who don't worry." He is telling her that at least some stress is universal. "Don't be so concerned about Tom."

But Sally continues to worry about Tom. She understands that when you are under stress a blockade is set up, preventing reinforcements (nutrients) from getting through. It's like pulling the emergency cord on a train. The response is immediate. Only one function matters. Everything else must come to a halt. When we are dealing with people, however, the ultimate consequence varies from individual to individual, depending in part on your own Achilles' heel. Sally was amused at how the variation of the stress effect is reflected in Tom's picturesque descriptions of symptoms:

"I felt as though fifty Boy Scouts were tying knots in my colon."

"A butterfly collection was let loose in my stomach."

"The Music Man's seventy-six trombones were parading in my head."

And a generalized feeling of stress: "Yesterday I spent a year doing routine office work."

The fact that different parts of the body are respondents of discomfort is further demonstrated when Tom assigns the affliction more to the source than the target:

"That business is a headache."

"She is a pain in the neck." (Or you know where else.)

"This report is blood, sweat, and tears."

And Tom, like everyone, views stress as an aging factor: "That took ten years off my life." Regardless of the ultimate manifestation of specific responses to stress, it all starts in Tom's brain: his hypothalamus defines an uncomfortable image, relaying this message to the networks, which in turn set up the barriers.

Table Talk: Stress

Sally explored the possibility of consuming those foods which supply in abundance the very nutrients that are wiped out by emotional stress. Tom, anticipating the minor plastic surgery, appeared to be ready for diet changes. Sally's findings:

- Acetylcholine is formed from choline, which is mostly extracted from ingested foods. As indicated, people under stress need increased amounts of acetylcholine. Isn't it interesting that acetylcholine levels increase in depression and decrease in mania?[30]

  Choline foods are: egg yolks, organ meats, brewer's yeast, whole grains, soy beans, fish, legumes, and lecithin.[31,32]

- When under stress, large amounts of ascorbic acid are lost, particularly from the adrenal cortex.[33] The intense breakdown induced by severe stress is also associated with loss of proteins, carbohydrates, and fats. The protein is lost because ascorbic acid is necessary for the manufacture of some of the amino acids (the building blocks of protein). Constituents of protein are not properly formed when ascorbic acid supplies are diminished.[34]

  Vitamin C rarely sets up permanent residency in the blood. Within a few hours, half the supply has vacated. If provisions were low to begin with, it may take up to twelve or thirteen hours to replenish, regardless of quantity ingested.[35] And why should supplies be depleted? Dr. Irwin Stone, world-renowned ascorbic acid researcher, says:

The human race has a genetic defect. We are missing an enzyme which is needed to produce ascorbic acid. A goat is about the same size as an average human being, and is therefore a good animal for comparison. When a goat is relaxed [and quietly grazing on tin cans and long-playing records], it will produce about thirteen grams of ascorbic acid per day. However, when stressed, the manufacture of ascorbic acid is increased to about one hundred or more grams. I believe that any human under any kind of stress will benefit greatly from increased intake of ascorbic acid.[36]

Ascorbic acid foods are: citrus fruit, rose hips, acerola cherries, alfalfa seeds, green vegetables, cantaloupe, strawberries, broccoli, tomatoes, green peppers.[37,38]

- At least a dozen studies have shown that serotonin precursors improve mood disorders.[39] (A precursor is a substance from which another substance is made.) Serotonin is a chemical messenger which transmits impulses between brain cells.[40] We begin to wonder what came first, chicken or egg: serotonin levels are lower in brains of people who are depressed.[41] In any case, if adequate quantities of amino acids are not available, then the manufacture of serotonin is impaired.[42] Tryptophan, a very important amino acid, is a significant precursor of serotonin. Tryptophan is necessary for the manufacture of serotonin.

  Foods containing tryptophan are: nuts and seeds, organ meats, brown rice, carrots, beets, celery, endive, dandelion greens, fennel, snap beans, brussel sprouts, chives, alfalfa.[43,44]

- Stress of any kind depletes the body of zinc.[45] In some people, stress causes urine excretion of a substance called kryptopyrrole, which takes with it both zinc and vitamin B_6.[46]

  Zinc foods are: sunflower seeds, seafood, organ meats, mushrooms, brewer's yeast, soybeans, eggs, whole grains.[47,48] Vitamin B_6 foods are: yeast, whole grains, organ meats, egg yolks, legumes, green leafy vegetables, desiccated liver, muscle meats.[49,50]

- The metabolic effects of chromium deficiency are greatly exaggerated in animals subjected to stress. One of these effects mimics that of insulin deficiency.[51]

  Chromium foods are: clams, whole grains, brewer's yeast.[52]

- Is it any wonder that people under stress are so tired? Stress often causes the urinary excretion of acids which chelate (grab) iron and other metals, removing them from the body.[53]

  Foods containing iron are: organ meats, egg yolks, fish, oysters, clams, whole grains, beans, green vegetables, desiccated liver.[54]

- We have already learned that the adrenal gland handles emotional stress via hormone regulation. Pantothenic acid supports this gland. When pantothenic acid-deficient diets are served to test subjects, they quickly become emotionally upset, irritable, quarrelsome, sullen, depressed, and dizzy.[55]

Foods containing pantothenic acids are: organ meats, brewer's yeast, eggs, legumes, sweet potatoes, whole grains, salmon.

• Among the consequences of having too many free fatty acids in your blood (as a result of stress) is the reduction of magnesium.[56] Magnesium is also lost as a result of the hormones secreted under stress. These same hormones interfere with the cellular magnesium/calcium ratio. A point of interest is that magnesium protects the arterial lining from the *mechanical* stresses caused by sudden changes in blood pressure.[57]

Magnesium is an element of power. One medical nutritionist, upon discovering that his magnesium level was dangerously low, reported that it took him five years to raise it to a respectable level. According to his statement, "achieving normal magnesium status demanded the cessation of smoking, curtailing the use of caffeine-containing beverages, giving up the social cocktail, and learning how to handle stress."[58]

Magnesium foods are: vegetables, whole grains, raw dried beans and peas, seafood, nuts.[59]

• Hormones secreted as a result of stress cause a decrease in the essential ratio of *potassium* and sodium on either side of the cell (within and without).[60]

Your body does make heroic attempts to defend itself against the negative effects of stress. ACTH, an adrenal hormone released under stress, in turn is responsible for the release of substances which increase blood pressure needed to cope with stress.[61] It accomplishes this mission by encouraging the retention of sodium and the excretion of potassium. This results in water retention, the consequence of which may be hypertension. Increased circulating blood fluid is one of the most dangerous aspects of hypertension.[62]

All ☆**natural foods**☆ contain more potassium than sodium—even those foods that are high in sodium. Food processing often reverses this ratio by decreasing potassium and adding salt. For example, a portion of fresh peas contains about 1 milligram of sodium and 380 milligrams of potassium. Your cells like it this way. Canned peas of equal size contain 230 milligrams of sodium and only 180 milligrams of potassium.[63] This is a set-up for malfunction. Your cells begin to scream out, "*Cannot compute,*" and if there is enough reason to protest, some cells see their final hour.

Potassium foods are: lean meats, whole grains, vegetables, legumes, sunflower seeds, bananas.[64]

* * *

Sally has enjoyed transforming this information into table talk. She found herself saying to a friend, with authority and assuredness, "If you are under stress, and you do not attempt to make the necessary life-style changes, it's Catch-22: stress causes malnourishment, and malnourishment causes stress."

JANE AND JIM TUNE IN

Nutrients Instead of Drugs

Jim's mother and grandmother had a favorite guru: a man giving nutrition advice on the radio for over forty years. Their devotion to this nutrition educator was the target of teasing until Jane's and Jim's newly cultivated interest in the subject. Dr. Carlton Fredericks has introduced the value of better eating to more people than any other human being.

Jane and Jim are part of a new generation of listeners. On the subject of stress, they learned from Dr. Fredericks that "more than forty-five years ago vitamin E was described as 'dampening the transmission of anxiety impulses from the thalamus (emotional brain) to the cortex (thinking brain).' "

Dr. Fredericks discusses other calming nutrients used in supplemental form:

. . . there is inositol, a factor of the vitamin ☆B complex☆, which has a quieting effect on the brain which, displayed on an electroencephalograph, is curiously close to that of tranquilizers, minus the side effects. Pantothenic acid, also a B complex factor, may be used for its action in helping the body better to tolerate stress. . . . Niacinamide, which acts upon the same cell receptors as do tranquilizers, quiets some individuals.

When vitamin C is to be administered, the nutritionist will also give bioflavonoids, factors that accompany ascorbic acid in foods and help its actions in the body.[65]

Additional information on the importance of niacin is demonstrated in the results of a study conducted in Sweden. Volunteer subjects were placed under stress, and as expected, fatty acids, triglycerides, heart rate, and blood pressure increased. A control group, exposed to the same stress, was given three grams of niacin. In this group, the fatty acids and triglyceride levels were reduced. (The other factors rose.)[66]

Jane and Jim also know that their exercise program is a fantastic stress reducer.

KEITH TRIES

=====================================

Learning to Control the Uncontrollable

Keith read a book on stress. Since he wasn't making much progress in his attempts to supply nutrients which are depleted during times of stress, he thought he might begin to examine other methods of stress-relieving activities. He learned that in addition to exercise, other modalities are encouraged for those people who no longer shift at will into the parasympathetic mode of behavior. He wasn't sure this applied to him, but the book was fascinating. Keith read that on-going high arousal states are primarily responsible for ultimate cellular disarray. Constant excitation could be replaced with a more calming and controlling body chemistry with the cultivation of skills which encourage low arousal. These include biofeedback, progressive relaxation methods, autohypnosis, and exercise (Keith's favorite), among others. One can acquire knowledge enabling the regulation of body activities which may have been totally automatic before now.

Dr. Charles Stroebel, in his book *QR: The Quieting Reflex*, describes a six-second technique for coping with stress anytime, anywhere. Although the mastery of the method may take up to six months, its application, once acquired, matches the speed of computer responses. Part of the training program involves conjuring up this image:

Imagine that you are climbing aboard your own very safe spaceship. Feel your body sitting down in the control chair. After getting comfortable, imagine the objects in your spaceship. You are taking off. You are beginning to feel the increasing gravity. You feel the pressure against you. Your body is tense. Grip the arms of your chair to brace against the force of gravity. Inhale a deep breath. Hold it. Your whole body is getting more and more tense. Tighten your toes, feet, and legs. Tighten your fingers, arms, and shoulders. Tighten your neck and face. Hold on! You are tight and tense; the gravity is increasing; the tension is growing harder and tighter. Now as you suddenly burst through the gravity field, exhale deeply. You're weightless. Your whole body loosens. Let your jaw, tongue, and shoulders go loose. Let your eyes smile. Let your neck and shoulders go loose. Your arms and fingers go limp. Your abdomen, thighs, and legs go loose. Your ankles, feet, and toes are heavy and loose and warm. Feel your muscles letting go as you float. Your body is weightless and safe. You feel serene. Say to yourself, "Alert mind, effortless body." Notice how you feel when your muscles let go, when you feel calm and serene. Your body has now floated safely back to where you began. You feel heavy, safe, and calm. Your body is sinking deeper and deeper into your chair. You feel heavy and calm. Stay completely motionless. Without actually doing it, think about lifting up one leg. Think about the muscles that you would have to use if you would have to raise your arm. Notice the tensions that have crept into these muscles just because of your thoughts. Thoughts can invade your muscles to make you feel tense or to make you feel calm.[67]

This is one exercise of many that eventually take the reader to the six-second *Quieting Response*. Keith was impressed. He thought he might give this a whirl. One of these days. Maybe.

It was an especially beautiful morning. Bob, as usual, was diagnosing. He noticed that "Handsome Guy" looked pale. What kind of stress was he under? Or was it stress? Hans Selye came to mind. Stress is not the cause of the alarm going off. It is the stressor that does that. And that depends on how you read the world around you. A favorite Selye anecdote sifted through:

Two young boys were raised by an alcoholic father. As they grew older, they moved away from that broken home, each going his own way in the world. Several years later, they happened to be interviewed separately by a psychologist who was analyzing the effects of drunkenness on children in broken homes. His research revealed that the two men were strikingly different from each other. One was a clean-living teetotaler, the other a hopeless drunk like his father. The psychologist asked each of them why he developed the way he did, and each gave an identical answer: "What else would you expect when you have had a father like mine?"[68]

For the best of all worlds, mused Bob, it's a combination of eating live food, exercising, and knowing how to handle stress. Not everyone on this track had that total prescription. But as a bunch, things were looking better.

"Old Guy" was moving faster than ever. He had told Bob that he had just become a great-grandfather, and that gave him extra energy today.

That cute young couple were running neck and neck and talking up a storm as they circumnavigated the track.

"Dumpy" was slimming down and looking younger. She had company now. Her husband? Was that why she was smiling? (Sally was smiling because her bra straps kept slipping off her shoulders, a direct result of having lost weight.)

The walking couple moved so fast, they almost kept up with the slow runners.

Even the dogs appeared to have boundless energy today. One of them scurried past Keith. Keith plunged forward, pushing himself as though in competition with the four-legged jogger. A sharp pain in his chest arrested the contest. He stopped, reeled, and collapsed.

Bob administered on-the-spot emergency measures while Jane and Jim ran to a phone to call for an ambulance. The others gathered around, waiting to be of assistance if necessary.

When it was over, the shock of the incident was somewhat softened for the aerobnics: Bob, Ben, Sally and Tom, and Jane and Jim watched Mike and Meg leave hand in (very close) hand.

Louis Pasteur says it his way: "The microbe is nothing; the terrain is everything."

CHAPTER 6

Specifics for the Pursuit of Youth

Mr. Jones complained to his doctor that he wasn't feeling very well, and that even his sex life was suffering. The doctor gave him a specific diet. In addition, he told him to walk ten miles a day and call him in a week. A week later Mr. Jones called the doctor.

"Well, Doc, I'm doing everything you said."

"Are you feeling better? Has your sex life improved?"

"I don't know," answered Jones, "I'm seventy miles from home."

OPTIMAL DIET FOR THE PURSUIT OF YOUTH

We have found the fountain of youth! No remote hidden pocket of the universe. No high-tech drug compounds. *The real fountain of youth is in your very own kitchen.*

It has been said that the doctor should care more for the individual patient than for the special features of the disease. This implies knowing a patient well enough to determine, among other things, whether food and life-style changes should be implemented quickly or at snail's pace, and that the specifics of a disease are not the most important considerations in cure.

Based on clinical experience at The Stress Center in Huntington, L.I., N.Y., we discovered that "optimal diet" could alleviate varied and sundry symptoms, mild or intense. Those who followed its tenets not only began to be free of symptoms, but looked incredibly younger.

"My internist told me that my multiple sclerosis was something I had to live with. He says it's pure coincidence that I look and feel so much better. I cannot convince him that it's the diet change."

"You mean it was that simple? I've been taking stool softeners for twenty years, since age thirteen, and in three weeks my problem has disappeared."

"For the first time in my life I have color in my face."

"For the first time in years I don't need an antacid after every meal."[1]

These are just a few of several hundred comments typical of those heard by medical nutritionists day after day. As for the tempo at which a person makes the changes, there are surprises. Some people don't want to get well—ever. Others with serious degenerative disease can only alter things slowly, even when more rapid modifications might mean quicker recovery. Those who give you the impression that you are wasting both your time and theirs during an initial counseling session, return in a week to report that they've made the changes "fell swoop." Personality and nutrition awareness, rather than degree of illness, dictate how receptive people are to turning things around.

Optimal diet appears stringent at first glance. But volumes have been filled with endless varieties of recipes based on the accepted foods.

Here it is:

You should not eat or drink:

NO!	*milk (whole), milk (skim or low fat), half-and-half, tea, coffee, de-caf, tap water, cheese and other milk prod-*	NO!
NO!	*ucts, fruit juice, head or iceberg lettuce, salt butter, margarine, dried fruit, citrus fruit, ice cream, pretzels,*	NO!
NO!	*canned soup, potato chips, wheat products, wheat germ, bran, white bread, white rice, supermarket whole wheat*	NO!
NO!	*bread, bottled oils, nuts purchased without shells (un-less sprouted), cola, diet soda, cake, cookies, crackers,*	NO!
NO!	*canned or frozen anything, sugar, salt, honey, pro-cessed flour.*	NO!

What's left?

You can eat:

    eggs (fertile only; poached, boiled, or sunny-side-up are best)
    sweet butter (in very small amounts)

these whole grains: millet, brown rice, buckwheat—with cinnamon or Eugalan Forte, but no milk
Essene bread (made from sprouted grains)
small amount of viable yogurt or acidophilus with each meal (2
tablespoons)
cold-water fish (eat the skin too)

You *must* eat:

vegetables—vegetables—vegetables—a lot! a lot! a lot! EVERY
DAY . . . A LOT! Raw. Lightly steamed. Raw. As much as the
appetite and digestion tolerate. You cannot overdose on vegetables. Leafy greens: parsley, watercress, bib or romaine lettuce, etc.

You can also eat:

fruit in moderation
Fruit formula: 1 fruit to 3 portions of vegetables (or 2 to 6). First,
eat 3 portions of vegetables. Then you may have one fruit, pref-
erably an apple.
condiments—all kinds; onions and garlic are excellent

You should eat: foods to reduce toxic levels (especially for city folk):

1 cup peas or beans daily (string beans, green peas, lentils, etc.)
1 cup alfalfa sprouts daily
lots of raw vegetables

Beverages

If herb teas are unpalatable, add unprocessed apple juice until taste
buds are reeducated. Diminish juice until it is no longer needed.
Add cinnamon or cinnamon stick to herb tea.
Drink lots of water (pure, of course).

Especially good foods

bananas (if no low blood sugar), lima beans, sweet potatoes, avocados, vegetable broths (homemade), millet, brewer's yeast, liver
and other organ meats, tempeh and tofu, homemade vegetable
blends, deep sea fish, sunflower seeds (purchased in the shell, unsalted, unroasted)

Some people respond to the diet changes immediately. Others require several months before feeling better. There are those who even
feel worse before improving. But there is a pot of gold at the end of
this rainbow.[2]

MENU PLAN FOR MILK- AND WHEAT-
INTOLERANTS

Recent studies indicate that celiac is never outgrown. Anyone who had problems with milk or wheat as an infant or child should consider a milk-free and wheat-free diet as an adult. These sensitivities are more widespread than most people (including physicians) realize. But it's easy to say to someone, "Don't consume any foods with wheat or milk." Not so easy, though, to carry this through. In answer to patients' requests (and complaints) at the Stress Center, we devised the following seven-day menu and recipe food plan:[3]
The basic tenets of good health are:

1. variety of healthful foods as outlined
2. quality (not necessarily quantity) protein with every meal
3. quality fiber with every meal

DAY 1
Breakfast: 2 poached eggs; rice cakes with butter; apple
Lunch: lentil soup;[a*] large salad[b]
Dinner: liver slivers;[c] lots of lightly steamed vegetables[d]

DAY 2
Breakfast: soy pancakes;[e] small banana
Lunch: tarator soup;[f] large salad[b]
Dinner: steamed chicken (organic);[g] lots of lightly steamed vegetables[d]

DAY 3
Breakfast: millet with cinnamon and banana slices[h]
Lunch: chicken salad;[i] Essene bread
Dinner: broiled fish;[j] lots of lightly steamed vegetables[d]

DAY 4
Breakfast: 2 eggs, sunny-side-up; grated carrot[k]
Lunch: string bean mousse;[l] large salad[b]
Dinner: oriental brown rice;[m] lots of lightly steamed vegetables[d]

* Recipes follow Day 7.

DAY 5
Breakfast: buckwheat pancakes with apples[n]
Lunch: tofu omelet;[o] large salad[b]
Dinner: salmon trout;[p] lots of lightly steamed vegetables[d]

DAY 6
Breakfast: avocado omelet[q]
Lunch: fish salad;[r] large salad[b]
Dinner: the "Soup"[s]

DAY 7
Breakfast: granola (wheat- and milk-free)[t]
Lunch: egg foo yung with tofu;[u]
Dinner: curried rice;[v] lots of lightly steamed vegetables[d]

Everyday staples: sunflower seeds (purchased unhulled, unsalted); raw
vegetables for nibbling; vegetable juices or blends (carrots, celery,
greens); small quantity of whole-milk yogurt, or Eugalan Forte, or
acidophilus with each meal
Everyday options: herb tea

Recipes

a. **Lentil Soup**
  ¼ cup olive oil
  2 medium onions, diced
  2 stalks celery, diced
  6 cups water
  1 cup lentils, rinsed
  8 oz tomato sauce
  2 cloves garlic, minced
  Freshly ground pepper to taste

Pour olive oil into large skillet and sauté onions and celery until
translucent. Add lentils to 6 cups water. Add tomato sauce, garlic,
pepper, sautéd onions, and celery. Stir. Bring to boil. Cover. Simmer
on low heat 1¼ hours. This soup can be prepared ahead—even the
day before. Add nitrite-free franks to soup if desired. (Serves 4 to 6)

b. **Salad**
A salad is an incongruous, heterogeneous, or haphazard mixture.
Based on this true definition of a salad, no two salads should be iden-

tical. Salads for the pursuit of youth contain at least six ingredients. Mix and match:

leafy green lettuce, parsley, watercress, red and/or green pepper, grated carrot, onion, green peas, grated or diced zucchini, cabbage, garlic, sunflower seeds, avocado, cucumbers, broccoli, asparagus, sesame seeds, endive, arugula and sprouts. No other food is as nutrient dense as home-grown sprouts. Add to the salad: alfalfa sprouted, radish, wheatberry, red clover, mung, chick-peas, rye, sunflower, lentil, azuki. (See Sprouting Instructions in the Appendix.)

c. Liver Slivers
½ lb liver
½ onion, sliced thin
Butter or oil
1 apple, spliced thin

Slice liver into thin, spaghetti-sized strands. Simmer onions in butter or oil; add liver and apple slices. Stir-fry quickly, moving pieces about while cooking. Do not overcook. This is a fast process. (Serves 1 or 2)

d. Steamed Vegetables
If you do not have a large steamer pot, buy an inexpensive steamer basket that makes a steamer of any pot you own with a cover. Steam only until vegetables reach prime color—still crisp. Slice those vegetables which cook quickly into thick pieces (zucchini, etc.); cut smaller chunks of slower cooking varieties (squash, sweet potato, etc.). Steam:

broccoli, squash, cabbage, zucchini, string beans, onion, brussel sprouts, sweet potato, peppers, green peas.

e. Soy Pancakes
3 eggs
4 tablespoons soy flour
1 cup hot water
Oil for pan
Lemon juice and mashed fruit for topping

Blend eggs and soy flour until smooth and thick. Put in bowl and stir in enough hot water to make thin batter. Transfer to pitcher. Brush hot pan with oil and pour in enough batter to make thin pancake.

Brown on both sides; fold in two. Set cooked pancake aside on hot plate until cool. Serve with mixed lemon juice and mashed fruit. (Serves 2)

f. **Tarator Soup**
 4 oz shelled walnuts
 5 peeled garlic cloves
 5 teaspoons olive oil
 5 cups plain yogurt
 ½ cup cold water
 1 medium-sized cucumber, peeled and diced
 Fresh parsley or dill

Mix walnuts and garlic. Add olive oil, a few drops at a time, stirring constantly, until smooth. In bowl, beat yogurt until smooth. Blend in walnut and garlic mixture and ½ cup of cold water. Add cucumber. Chill in refrigerator. Serve cold, sprinkled with finely chopped parsley or dill. This is the best cold soup you've ever eaten. (Serves 6)

g. **Steamed Chicken**
 1 small organic chicken
 1 teaspoon oregano
 2 cloves garlic, minced
 ½ teaspoon paprika

Place chicken in steamer basket over an inch or two of water. Bring water to boil. Steam on low heat for 30 minutes, covered. Remove chicken, cut into eighths. Dust with oregano and sprinkle with garlic and paprika. Broil until golden brown. (Serves 3 or 4)

h. **Easy Millet**
 1 cup water
 ½ cup millet
 Cinnamon
 Banana, sliced

Boil water. Add millet. Lower heat and cook, covered, 15 to 20 minutes, or until all water is absorbed. Add dash of cinnamon and sliced banana. (Serves 1 or 2)

i. **Chicken Salad**
   Last night's leftover chicken
   1 stalk celery
   Seasonings to taste
   Homemade mayonnaise

   Dice chicken; add celery and seasonings and mayonnaise to taste.

j. **Broiled Fish**
   1 green pepper
   1 small onion
   1 clove garlic
   ½ teaspoon minced ginger
   Butter or oil for pan
   Fresh fish from deep ocean
   ½ cup sesame seeds
   Juice of ½ lemon
   Parsley for trim

   Simmer pepper, onion, garlic, and ginger in butter or oil. Place fish on top, and simmer for about 10 minutes. Sprinkle sesame seeds on top, and place under broiler until done. Add lemon juice. Garnish with crushed parsley. (Serves 2)

k. **Grated Carrot**
   2 small or 1 big carrot, grated
   ½ onion
   Sprouted sunflower seeds.

   Combine all. (Serves 2)

l. **String Bean Mousse**
   2 cups lightly steamed string beans
   2 hard cooked eggs
   2 tablespoons homemade mayonnaise
   Garlic and seasonings to taste

   Toss all ingredients into food processor (or blender) and whip until light and frothy. (Eggbeater is okay too.) (Serves 2 to 4)

m. **Oriental Brown Rice**
   1 tablespoon sesame oil
   1 cup brown rice

2½ cups water
1 cup mushrooms
2 cups bean sprouts
1 cup green peas
1 cup chopped scallions
1 cup diced water chestnuts
1 cup chopped celery
1 cup chopped green or red pepper
4 cloves mashed garlic
3 additional tablespoons sesame oil
1 teaspoon tamari
2 eggs

Place 1 tablespoon oil in skillet and heat. Add rice slowly, with heat still on, stirring continuously until each grain is coated with oil. This takes only a few minutes, but prevents grains from sticking. Pour water into another pot. Bring to boil. Add oil-coated rice slowly and cover pot. Reduce heat to lowest possible setting. Cook 30 minutes. (No peeking; don't let the steam out.) Stir-fry mushrooms quickly; set aside. Add remainder of ingredients, except eggs and tamari. Stir-fry quickly. Add tamari. Add rice and stir all. Lightly scramble 2 eggs; toss into mix. Optional: add 1 or 2 cups diced chicken or turkey (only if organic). (Serves 4)

n. **Buckwheat Pancakes**
2 eggs
2½ cups buttermilk
2 tablespoons butter
2 cups buckwheat flour
1½ teaspoons baking power (aluminum-free variety)
Whole-milk yogurt

Combine eggs and buttermilk. Add butter, and beat mix thoroughly. In separate container, stir together flour and baking powder, pressing out any lumps. Add liquid ingredients, stirring only until blended. Add water if too thick; more flour if too thin. Drop batter on slightly greased hot griddle. Cook until just a bit dry on top (bubbles will form); turn and cook on other side. Serve hot. Serve with yogurt. (Serves 4 to 6)

o. **Tofu Omelet**
Butter for pan

1 green pepper, diced
½ cake tofu
½ cup mushrooms, diced
1 small onion, diced
5 eggs, beaten
Alfalfa sprouts

Melt butter in pan. Simmer pepper, tofu, mushrooms, and onions in butter. Add beaten eggs. Stir while cooking until eggs are done. Serve with alfalfa sprouts. (Serves 2 or 3)

p. **Salmon Trout**
This fish is so good as is, all it requires is broiling with a little bit of butter and pressed fresh garlic.

q. **Avocado Omelet**
Butter for pan
2 eggs, beaten
¼ avocado

Heat pan with butter; pour in beaten eggs. Let eggs cook pancake style. Add diced avocado to one-half of pancake egg, folding over second half. Allow to heat through. (Serves 1)

r. **Fish Salad**
Last night's left-over fish
Seasonings

Mix with seasonings as desired.

s. **The Soup**
2 quarts water
½ cup rice (or barley or millet)
½ cup each: diced onion, green pepper, celery, carrot, sweet potato, zucchini squash, mushrooms
Dash pepper
Clove crushed garlic
Oregano, dried
Thyme, dried
Basil, dried
1 tablespoon tamari

Bring water to boil. Add rice (or other grain). Reduce heat and cover. Cook over low heat for ½ hour. Add vegetables, seasonings, and tamari. Barely simmer for 1 to 2 hours, or until ready to eat.

t. **Granola** (Wheat- and Milk-free)
rice flakes, raisins, toasted soy nuts, pecans, rice flour, honey, oil, water, vanilla

Experiment. Mix and match to taste.

u. **Egg Foo Yung With Tofu**
1 cup alfalfa sprouts (or mixture of sprouts)
3 eggs, lightly beaten
6 ounces tofu, cut into small squares
½ green pepper, thinly sliced
¼ cup minced onion
1 teaspoon tamari
4 teaspoons oil
Pepper

Combine first six ingredients, mixing well. Heat 2 teaspoons oil in heavy skillet. Pour in one half of egg/tofu mixture to form thin omelet. Cook for 2½ minutes on each side until nicely browned. Repeat until all ingredients have been used. Top with pepper. (Serves 2 to 4)

v. **Curried Rice**
2 tablespoons butter
1 medium onion, chopped
1 apple, cored and chopped
½ cup raisins (soaked)
2 cups cooked brown rice
Curry powder to taste
2 tablespoons chopped peanuts

Heat butter in saucepan. Sauté onion, apple, and raisins until tender. Add rice and mix. Stir in curry powder. Garnish with peanuts.
Variations: Use millet instead of rice; almonds or coconut instead of peanuts. (Serves 4 to 6)

FOR THOSE WHO WORK: SOME OF THESE LUNCHES CAN BE PREPARED THE NIGHT BEFORE.

If we do not put the effort into health, we often have to put it into sickness. [3]

LISTEN TO YOUR BODY

Keeping a food diary can be very revealing. You might discover that the headache you get on occasion occurs two days after you had hot chocolate. Or that the feeling of extreme fatigue happens the evening of your lunch date with your mother-in-law. (It could be your mother-in-law, or the Bloody Mary you have before you meet her.) Maybe the arthritis flares up when you have two or three pieces of bread. Your cravings may have a pattern too!

Here's an outline for a food diary:

Food Diary

Note: list specific ingredients of salads and vegetable platters. Indicate any food that was canned, frozen, eaten in a restaurant, or commerically prepared and brought home.

Breakfast:

Morning Snacks:

Lunch:

Afternoon Snacks:

Dinner:

Evening Snacks:

Midnight Refrigerator Raids:

Glasses of water today:

Supplements taken today:

# of cigarettes smoked today:

Time spent with others smoking today:

Drugs taken today (medical):

Drugs taken today (recreational, including caffeine and alcohol):

Were you constipated today?

Did you have diarrhea today?

Did you sleep well last night?

Any other distresses today?

Specific time(s) of day you felt particularly good:

Specific time(s) of day you felt particularly bad:

What percent of vegetables consumed today were raw:

What percent of vegetables consumed today were cooked:

How many foods consumed today were not whole, natural foods?

What kind of salad dressing, if any, did you use today?

What condiments did you use today?

Did you find it difficult to consume only healthful foods today?

You don't have to be a trained diagnostician to see patterns if you have kept an accurate diary. Try it—it works! And then share your discoveries with your medical nutritionist.

CONSTIPATION

Constipation is almost always the result of improper diet. High fiber often solves the problem. Although bran has the highest fiber content of any food product, it is far better to obtain fiber from whole, natural foods. The usual consequences occur when we change the architecture of an edible substance. Bran as sold separately is the outer coating of a grain (usually that of wheat or oats). Wheat bran has been shown to raise cholesterol slightly, and any grain bran has been shown to delete minerals.

If you do use bran as a constipation remedy, be sure to soak the bran overnight, or at least for several hours, and take the bran with liquid (a glass of water).

Possible causes of constipation are:

iron supplements
over-refined and starchy foods (white bread, white rice, bakery products)
hard-cooked eggs
cheese
meat
boiled milk
hot drinks
foods containing tannin (red wine, tea, cocoa)
cloves
pasta

To reduce constipation, try:

foods that absorb moisture readily (celery, radishes, carrots, lettuce)
foods that are slightly laxative (raw figs, raw spinach, strawberries, sesame seeds, watermelon)
lots of fluids
☆**herbs and other high-nutrient foods**☆
garlic (prescribed by Hippocrates for constipation)
dandelion leaf tea
psyllium and flax seeds
brewer's yeast
rice polishings

☆**high fiber foods**☆
> millet, wheat, rice, barley, rye, buckwheat,
> peas, beans, lentils, nuts (chewed well), seeds,
> potatoes, carrots, parsnips, turnips,
> leafy vegetables, cabbage, celery

These high fiber foods have been listed in order of fiber excellence. That is, grains have more fiber than legumes, which have more fiber than root vegetables, which have more fiber than leafy vegetables.

Two effective recipes are:

1. dried prunes soaked overnight in water with lemon juice
2. a blend of 1 tablespoon of pumpkin seeds, 2 ounces of sesame seeds, 1 cup of soaked raisins. Add enough warm water to make one quart; sip throughout the day.

Try grating a raw carrot into your salad—daily.

Most *primary* foods are high-fiber foods. People on high-fiber diets (☆whole foods☆) rarely suffer from constipation.[4,5]

MENSTRUATION DIFFICULTIES

Do not accept menstrual difficulties as normal just because they are average. You can turn things around: you can reduce heavy flows, you can cut down on the length of time of the period, and you do not have to experience severe or even mild discomfort once a month. Menstrual difficulties are signs of imbalance. Imbalance is not a plus factor in your pursuit of youth.

- Heavy periods can be due to a shift in hormone levels. Sometimes irregular periods are promoted because of sudden weight loss (crash diets) or extreme emotional stress. Obesity, on the other hand, can cause irregular cycles and increased blood loss.
- Undernutrition delays the onset of menstruation and interferes with regulation. Fat stores are possible energy stores for hormone production.
- One to three pounds are often gained prior to menstruation, and lost as soon as the period starts. When premenstrual tension is

present, the body stores a greater amount of salt and water just before the menstrual flow starts. A temporary imbalance between estrogen and progesterone takes place. Breast tenderness can be caused by fluid retention and altered hormone levels.

- Iron losses during menstruation are constant for each woman, but vary from woman to woman. Inadequate iron levels are due to inadequate iron intake—not menstruation. Iron foods are: dark green leafy vegetables, whole grains, liver and other organ meats, and shellfish.
- Ascorbic acid is lowest during menstruation, so supplementation is indicated. Another study shows that women taking B_6 and zinc had normal cycles within three months.
- B-vitamins and protein are needed by the liver to convert hormones necessary for the menstrual process. Bioflavonoids were shown to be helpful. Depression subsides with B_6 in some cases.
- Childbirth helps because it stretches the cervical canal. Also, there are fewer contractions with each period once you have had a baby.
- There are two types of dysmenorrhea—hypercontractability of the muscles of the uterus can occur in the absence of disease or can be disease related. Primary dysmenorrhea is discomfort that has no known reason. *Dys* means discomfort and *menorrhea* applies to the flow of the period.

Part of the pain is due to the presence of hormone-like substances called prostaglandins, which are present in higher levels if dysmenorrhea is present. That is why traditional doctors give prostaglandin inhibiting drugs. But of course dysmenorrhea is a sign that something is out of balance. There are several families of prostaglandins, and only one type (in raised levels) causes the problem. Inhibiting drugs, however, depress all types.

Prostaglandins were first identified in prostate tissue, and later in menstrual fluid. They stimulate the contraction of the uterine smooth muscle. So they were called menstrual stimulants. Women with pain have higher levels of prostaglandins, and different ratios of different types. The discomfort may have to do with high prostaglandin levels and/or their metabolites which are involved with the contractability of muscle tissue. It may also have to do with not having enough good blood circulation to the uterus organ itself.

Women with higher levels of prostaglandins may have higher levels of certain types of estrogen, called estradiol. Liver functioning has a lot to do with the amount of estradiol in the body. Lipotrophic factors (which aid fat metabolism) are essential for proper liver functioning, i.e., "optimal diet."

Certain trace minerals can decrease the inflammatory contractile characteristic of the prostaglandins: copper and zinc. Magnesium and B_6, a powerful vitamin hormone regulator, are also recommended.

In addition, unsaturated fatty acids are helpful. If you are a good responder and absorb fatty acids well, eating foods that contain these acids will suffice (avocados, sunflower seeds, and other nuts and seeds). If you are a poor responder, the use of one of the most powerful unsaturated fatty acids is advised: gamma linolenic acid.[6]

At the Department of Gynecology at St. Thomas's Hospital Medical School in London, sixty-eight women with severe premenstrual syndrome were treated with gamma linolenic acid. Almost complete relief of symptoms was seen in 62 percent, and partial relief in 22 percent. The average dose administered was two capsules twice daily from three days before expected onset of symptoms until the start of menstruation. Excellent results were obtained with premenstrual breast discomfort. Mood changes, fluid retention, and headache were also improved.[7]

Few foods contain any substantial amount of gamma linolenic acid. It is found in human milk, in a wild flower called the evening primrose, and in borage. (Borage is an herb unfamiliar to most Americans. In the sixteenth century borage had a reputation for making people happy! Today, the finely chopped leaves having a cucumber-like flavor are used with yogurt and cream cheese.) Gamma linolenic acid is available in supplemental form.

- In summary, reduce sodium intake (eliminate table salt, soy sauce, and processed foods); eat potassium-rich foods (bananas, almonds, avocados, cress, sesame and sunflower seeds); drink lots of water; eat a high bulk diet, whole grains and raw vegetables. Supplement with natural B-complex, such as brewer's yeast (especially absorbable in liquid form as Zell Oxygen); add calcium, magnesium, zinc, vitamin B_6, vitamin C, and gamma linolenic acid. One caution: several products labeled "Evening Primrose Oil" were tested and found to have virtually no gamma linolenic acid. The bottle you purchase should state clearly that it contains gamma linolenic acid (sometimes abbreviated GLA). This is the kind of essential fatty acid that will be therapeutic. This does not mean that other varieties are not authentic, but this notation is an assurance that you are getting the real stuff.[8]

While waiting for things to turn around, try back massage, hot pads, tub soaks, and rest to alleviate pain.

MENOPAUSE

Menopause is not a disease, nor is it abnormal. It is not something that should be stopped or delayed artificially. Rather than considered as negative, menopause should be viewed as a time of relief from fear of pregnancy.

Menopause is characterized by hot flashes and sweats. Since these symptoms yield to estrogen therapy, other symptoms are often regarded as those of instability. Symptoms other than these, however, are not necessarily psychological.

These symptoms can be avoided if one goes into menopause in good health. Several nutritional approaches are helpful:

- Vitamin E in large doses for sweats and flashes. Vitamin E antagonizes estrogen and thus indirectly improves thyroid balance. Vitamin E's therapeutic effects are widespread.
- Vitamin B_6 helps counteract edema. It is reported to aid in sulphur transport.
- Ginseng, garlic, onion, and cayenne pepper contain sulphur. This is the link between building blocks of most of the pituitary hormones.
- Ginseng's effects are enhanced when accompanied by vitamin E. Ginseng is also a pituitary regulator. Purchase in capsule form, unless you are certain of the source.
- Iodine, found in kelp and seafood, picks up thyroid function. It is best to secure iodine from these natural sources rather than in tablet form.
- Calcium, especially from dark green, raw, leafy vegetables, is helpful. Dairy products contain phosphorus in high amounts (so do meats), which tends to bind minerals such as calcium. Osteoporosis (reduction in the amount of calcium in the bone) causes the shorter and "dumpy" look of older women. This can be avoided if calcium

imbalances are avoided. There is a tendency to endocrine imbalance while the menopause transition is going on. Therefore, cut down on dairy products, and increase those dark green leafy vegetables. Cod-liver oil and magnesium are necessary for calcium absorption.

- Gamma linolenic acid has proved helpful. In fact, in five women who were one to three years postmenopausal and who were taking gamma linolenic acid for other reasons, regular menstrual cycles were restored. This is still experimental evidence, but we do know that a lack of this essential fatty acid could play a key role in the aging process in general. If menopause is reversible, other aging factors may also be reversible.[9]
- Parsley tea, watermelon, and cucumbers are good additions to the diet. So are gluten-free grains (millet and brown rice), and a preponderance of raw vegetables, raw seeds, and nuts.
- Exercise improves all body functions and should be included as an important part of this regimen.
- It should go without saying that all processed foods (anything in a can, carton, or box) should be eliminated. Sugar is the worst offender.

Pathological states are not normal just because they are prevalent. The management of menopause should be in the hands of self-reliant women. It is not a disease.[10]

★   ★   ★

It is best to consult with a good medical nutritionist before embarking on self-medication regimes. What you can do for yourself is exercise and follow "optimal diet."

★   ★   ★

With apologies to Oliver Wendell Holmes:

If all manufactured foods as now used could be sunk to the bottom of the sea, it would be all the better for humankind, and all the worse for fishes.

But then there's the story of the man who never ate one crumb of food other than natural. He lived an exemplary life-style. When he died and went to heaven, he was served celery and carrot sticks, but he noticed that "down there," in that other place, everyone was feasting on the most delectable gourmet foods. He complained to St. Peter.

"How come I've been given such meager pickings? Especially after my most exalted food selection through the years?"

St. Peter answered, "It doesn't pay to cook for two."

CHAPTER 7

Immunity and the Pursuit of Youth

The patient was sixty and his doctor advised that a man in his sixties shouldn't play tennis. He heeded the doctor's advice carefully and said he could hardly wait until he reached seventy to start again.

The Miracle of Immunity

The greatest miracle of all time is that we exist. The immune process which keeps us alive is part of that miracle. The fact that we are capable of understanding that immune process is another miracle. The air we breathe, the water we drink, the food we eat—all contain untold billions of microorganisms, viruses, pollutants, toxins, and as yet unidentified substances, many of which are lethal. How do we manage to keep these enemies at bay? We are alive to do more than speculate: our knowledge is extraordinarily sophisticated.

The body has functional and protective securities against these mischief-makers, enabling it to distinguish foreign material from self, and to neutralize, eliminate, or metabolize invaders. It does so by the physiologic mechanism of the immune response, the function of which is defense.

The thymus gland is the master gland of the immune system. We now know it produces important hormones involved in immune function (i.e., thymosin). It aids in the control of autoimmune disease (disease resulting from substances produced in the body which do damage to normal functions), and it helps control infectious diseases. It is also the site of T-cell production—the cells which fight and destroy bacteria, fungi, viruses, and mutated cells. As early as 1845 the thymus was described as a critical barometer of nutritional status.

Thymuses of undernourished children are consistently small and weigh less than one-half of a normal organ.[1] The thymus shrinks intensely under stress.[2] In 1936, Hans Selye proposed that in the "alarm reaction" due to stress of any kind (emotional, or stress caused by malnutrition), there is a direct negative effect on the thymus.[3] In one test study, animals fed on a protein-deficient diet of baker's flour for four months showed marked changes in thymus weight, so much so that no thymus could be detected in some of them.[4]

In addition to T-cells, there are other cells which promote immune responses. B-cells also produce antibodies which lead to the destruction of toxins and bacteria, and phagocytic cells engulf and destroy bacteria and other intruders.

The Looming Lymphatics

Lymph is the clear fluid that bathes all tissues of the body. The vessels that carry lymph also carry lymphocytes (a type of white blood cell) and other substances essential for the body's natural defense system—the immune process.[5]

It's easy to conjure up an image of your vascular system—that vast network of arteries, veins, and capillaries powered by an efficient, and sometimes noisy, but never resting heart. The heart pumps blood through this network to deliver nutrients and oxygen, and anything else needed (and sometimes a few things that are not needed). At the same time it also performs its sanitation engineering by removing toxins and waste products. But mention the lymph system, and you draw a blank. The lymph system just hasn't gotten as much P.R. or made as much commotion as the goings-on of the circulatory processes. But the lymph system parallels the vascular system in importance. It does its job modestly, without fanfare.

The lymph system is a secondary circulatory pathway that moves lymph fluid through every cell in your body. The lymphocytes it carries with it are like complex miniature computers. They recognize alien matter, and then present a blueprint to special plasma cells in order that the proper antibodies can be manufactured. These antibodies challenge and destroy potential troublemakers.

Lymph fluid is in no hurry. It moves through vessels slowly. When you are at rest, it would never get a speeding ticket. It travels at the rate of about four fluid ounces per hour. But watch out for the state troopers when you exercise: the lymph fluid speeds up by a factor of fifteen.

If exercise or moving about gets your immune system working faster and more efficiently, this seems to invalidate the concept of bed rest when you have an infection. The lymph fluid is a crucial cog in the get-well wheel. Muscular activity powers the lymph system, causing lymph vessels to compress and expand, to stretch and relax, which promotes movement of the vital lymph fluid. It's like squeezing the water out of a soft plastic container. (Another plus for daily ☆aerobics☆.)

Thixotrophy

If you ever put a cup of Jell-O on a vibrating surface, you have seen it turn to liquid very quickly. The fluid can become semisolid again. This phenomenon is called thixotrophy. "Thixis" is Greek for *touch*, and "tropos" is Greek for *a turning*. The protoplasm of your cells has thixotrophic properties—it can be "turned" to fluid with motion and activity, and turned back again to gel.

In the liquid state, the cellular protoplasm is able to absorb nutrients, discharge waste, and generally perform its biochemical miracles. When it is sedentary, it turns to gel, and all life processes slow down, making it more difficult for entry and exit of nutrients and toxins.

Does this mean we need to take up belly dancing to get our protoplasm shaking? Not necessarily. Walking a mile a day converts protoplasm to the state that will enhance biological activity. If no other exercise is possible, blow up balloons. Even that will help. (If you prefer the belly dancing, that's okay too.)

It should be emphasized that it is difficult to get a biological response from nutrients taken by mouth unless you are exercising.[6]

Exercise also induces perspiration, which is indicative of increased body temperature, another method for converting the protoplasm to a more liquid state. As Jell-O will liquefy at higher temperatures, so the cell protoplasm remains liquid when it is warmer.

Fever and Immunity

The recognition of fever as a sign of disease goes back at least as far as Hippocrates. Accurate observations were made with precise descriptions of the temperature course in many diseases. How this was done without benefit of Becton Dickinson remains a mystery. (Becton Dickinson manufactures all those fever thermometers.)

It is clear that fever is a regulated rise in body temperature at a time when the body needs added heat in the presence of infection. This encourages the immune system to work more efficiently in a liquid protoplasmic environment. It creates a milieu for the production of special infection fighting hormones.

Lizards do not have internal temperature controls. They modify their body temperature entirely by behavioral means. When infected, they seek warmer environments that raise their temperature, and their survival is directly correlated with the elevated temperature.[7]

In mammals, T-cell proliferation and antibody production increase when fever is present. Evolution appears to have given us the ability to stimulate vital defense mechanisms of cells against infection, and also to provide an optimal body temperature for these events to take place. Many researchers and physicians believe that we err when we attempt to reduce mild fever instead of letting it run its course.[8]

Manipulating Immunity

Just as organ reserve declines as we get older, so does immune competency. And, like organ reserve, some people appear to have more or less than average immune performance. In general, it decreases with age. It is possible that the slow progressive decline in immune response may be due to deficiencies of nutrients.

A single nutrient deficiency can result in profound impairment of specific immunologic processes. These immunologic defects resulting from even marginal deficiencies may affect the course of and/or response to disease. Nutrient deficiency is not an exclusive problem of underdeveloped countries. One study demonstrated that 88 percent of American patients examined had at least one deficiency, and 59 percent had two or more biochemical deficiencies. Before hospitalization, 61 percent had been eating what was considered a normal American diet.[9]

There is evidence that the immune imbalance of aging can be altered by dietary manipulations. These observations are fundamental in the pursuit of youth.[10] Examples:

- The most important immunologic effects produced by ☆**B-vitamins**☆ are seen with deficiencies of B$_6$, pantothenic acid, and folic acid.

1. Pyridoxine deficiency (B$_6$): consequences are poor antibody production after immunizations; decreased thymic hormone activity; impaired DNA and protein manufacture; and depression of cellular immunity.
2. Pantothenic acid deficiency: consequences are depressed antibody responses after immunizations.
3. Folic acid deficiency: depressed immune functions; atrophied lymphoid tissue.[11]

- ☆**Vitamin C**☆ is involved with overall cell health and protection. In particular, it must be present in adequate levels for proper production of interferon, the molecule that complexes with viruses and ultimately leads to their destruction. Vitamin C influences the healing of wounds. It decreases in the white blood cells during infections. Moderate doses have been shown to improve phagocytic function. (Phagocytes are cells that ingest foreign particles.)[12] As far back as 1939, the correlation between vitamin C and immunity was established. Administration of vitamin C to tuberculous guinea pigs increased the tolerance to repeated large doses of tuberculin.[13]
- Small increases in dietary ☆**vitamin A**☆ enhance resistance to infection in test animals and responsiveness to antigenic stimuli. (An antigen is an enemy substance to which the body reacts by producing antibodies.) Deficiency of vitamin A leads to depressed resistance to bacterial, viral, and protozoan infections.

Vitamin A maintains the composition of external cell membranes. Epithelial linings and mucous membranes of the body are the first sites penetrated by the invaders. Vitamin A is intimately involved with the maintenance of these tissues.

- Deficiencies of ☆**vitamin E**☆ depress general resistance. Increased amounts enhance the ability to survive experimental infections.
- Zinc, a ☆**trace mineral**☆, helps to regulate immune functions. It is essential for lymphocyte transformation and the defensive mecha-

nism against microorganisms.[14] Zinc is severely depleted during chronic infectious illnesses. Deficiency causes atrophy of lymphoid tissue. In severely zinc deficient animals, thymic hormone activity is depressed. It has been demonstrated that immune deficiencies can be reversed by restoring zinc.

- Stephen Levine, Ph.D., discusses an interesting concept in relation to ☆**selenium**☆:

The most critical of the antioxidant nutrients are antiinflammatory, and are the same nutrients that one finds as being most important for the immune response. Selenium has been used as an antiinflammatory agent by veterinarians for years. Selenium is known to improve antibody production and protect against cancer.[15]

- Abnormalities in lipid intake or metabolism can initiate important changes in immunity. ▫**Hypercholesterolemia**▫ (too much cholesterol) tends to decrease resistance to bacteria, viral infections, and tumors.[16] This is one example of abnormal lipid intake.

Another very significant example concerns essential fatty acid deficiency, which impacts on the immune system at the cellular level.

Is it any surprise that the ☆**positive**☆ antiaging substances listed in our compendium match those that mediate immunity, whereas the ▫**negatives**▫ are the very ones that reduce immune performance?

Optimizing Immunity

Dr. David Rowe, who is with the special program for research and training of the World Health Organization, says:

No doubt all nutritional problems could be solved by food, but unless we are so sanguine as to imagine that an optimal diet will in the near future be available for all, it would be well to consider possible strategies to minimize the adverse effects of malnutrition.[17]

If nutritional deficiency and susceptibility to disease through depressed immune activity go hand in hand, measures to stave off such deficiencies must be paramount in the pursuit of youth. Dr. Warren Levin, medical director of The World Health Medical Group, has prepared a special paper for this book offering his views on the pursuit of youth and how to optimize immunity, thereby potentiating longevity:

NUTRIENT SUPPLEMENTATION

The days of frank vitamin deficiency in the United States are pretty well past! Except for scattered cases found in schizophrenics, hermits, chronic severe alcoholics, and other truly unusual situations, the average person gets enough supplementation from cereals and "enriched" grain products so that beriberi and pellagra are now relics of the past.

There are, however, other major problems that are currently recognizable, but are not being searched out by the average practicing physician. I am referring to low-grade deficiency diseases of dietary fiber, macro- and micro-minerals, and essential fatty acids. Each of these is capable of contributing to less than optimum health, and when combined with the excesses of antinutrients—refined carbohydrates, hydrogenated fats, chemical pollutants, caffeine, alcohol, tobacco, insecticides, detergents (the list could go on and on)—could produce the nonspecific degenerative diseases of our Western "civilization." Correction of the problem calls for avoidance of these antinutrients and supplementation of those missing elements that we know about.

I want to state here a separate thought, which is intentionally capitalized: I believe that there are MULTIPLE UNKNOWN BUT STILL ESSENTIAL SYNERGISTIC MICRONUTRIENT COFACTORS THAT MAKE FOOD DIFFERENT FROM VITAMIN PILLS!!! Therefore, your first obligation as an intelligent consumer for good nutrition is to eat a great deal of fresh, wholesome food, carefully chosen and carefully prepared to preserve nutrient qualities. A wide variety is essential, and if, in so doing, you can calculate that you have achieved approximately the U.S. RDA for all of the known nutrients, you can then assume that you have probably obtained adequate quantities of the unknown factors.

Using ordinary store-bought food in the major metropolitan areas of this country today requires the consumption of at least 2,000 calories per day to achieve this goal! If you are one of those small people with a weight problem, you may recoil in horror, saying, "If I ate 2,000 calories I'd blow up to the size of a barn!" That does not change the reality of what your body needs in order to be healthy! What it means, then, is that you must increase your activity until you burn up enough calories so that you can eat enough good healthful food to give your body everything it requires to be well. There is no easy way out!

Now then, once you have eaten your 2,000 calories of healthful food, I then believe that supplementation will carry you from this minimum standard of nutrition represented by the United States Government's RDA to an optimum state which each of us should be aiming for in our personal quest for health and longevity. With that in mind, I propose the following supplementation program: a low potency ☆**B-complex**☆ vitamin formula based primarily according to guidelines propounded by Roger Williams, Ph.D.

B_1	(*thiamine*)	5 mg
B_2	(*riboflavin*)	5 mg
B_3	(*niacinamide*)	50 mg
B_5	(*pantothenic acid*	50 mg
B_6	(*pyridoxine*)	10 mg
B_{12}	(*cobalamin*)	25 mcg
PABA		100 mg

Other factors, such as choline and inositol, are loosely included in the B-complex. It is possible to obtain concentrated forms because they minimize the amount of fat and phosphate consumed in conjunction with essential factors. You should be able to get over 50 percent phosphatidyl choline and phosphatidyl inositol, combined with phosphatidyl ethanolamine. One heaping teaspoon of such a granular mixture should be more than adequate. But even this amount of phosphate needs to be consumed with care. If possible, any mineral supplementation should be taken at another time, to avoid an insoluble complex of mineral and phosphate residues, which may interfere with proper mineral absorption from the intestine.

There should no longer be any doubt about the importance of antioxidants in the roles of longevity and avoidance of degenerative disease. These nutrient factors have total scientific validation at the present time with regard to stabilizing the all-important membrane functions in every cell of the body. This prevents the submicroscopic damage to the cells themselves, which ultimately leads to impaired function at the cellular level—progressing to tissues and organs and finally to vital functions of the entire body.

The mechanism at work here is known technically as "free radical pathology." While it may not account for every degenerative problem, it is clearly a major factor in a number of varied presentations of chronic degenerative diseases. In addition, these antioxidants serve to protect against the conversion of precursors of carcinogenic substances into the actual carcinogen itself. (A specific example is the protection that vitamin C affords against the ingested nitrates which are converted in the body to carcinogenic substances known as nitrosamines.) My recommendations for these essential substances include:

Vitamin A	25,000 units per day
Beta carotene	25,000 to 50,000 units per day
Vitamin E	400 units (Preferably as mixed tocopherols. This is a minimum dose for patients who don't have problems with hypertension or rheumatic heart disease.)
Vitamin C	At least 3,000 milligrams per day
Bioflavonoids	500 milligrams per day
Glutathione	50 milligrams per day
Selenium	200 micrograms per day

Other nutrient factors that function in this antioxidant category are included elsewhere in the list. In addition, you may see recommendations for BHT and Ascorbyl Palmitate. These substances are both nonphysiologic and experimental, and although the results of preliminary studies are interesting, the regular use of such products represents an excessive extrapolation from limited facts. It would place anyone participating in such programs in an uncontrolled experimental therapeutic trial.

With regard to dietary fiber, it is generally true that a broad spectrum of healthful foods including the various complex carbohydrates such as whole grains, legumes, nuts, seeds, and fruits should provide adequate amounts.

Nevertheless, our total falls far short of many of the high fiber diets found in primitive cultures. I see no objection to the addition of dietary fiber as a supplement, with the understanding that "fiber" is a comprehensive term that should be called "the fiber complex" (similar to the B complex and C complex).

Overutilization of a single factor such as wheat bran exclusively may be good for bowel function, but probably is inappropriate in terms of other functions of fiber: adjustment of trace mineral balance, removal of toxic minerals, control of cholesterol and other fats, maintenance of proper intestinal flora, control of rate of absorption of macro- and micro-nutrients, and so on. It is more appropriate to supplement with a blend of various dietary fibers including, but not limited to, psyllium, alfalfa, pectin, cellulose, glucomannan, hemicellulose, lignin, algin, agar, and gums including guar, tragacanth, and karaya.

Those reading this book are obviously interested in the question of longevity and are much more likely than the average individual to look at other books on the subject. Many opinions are currently being promulgated about nutrition and life extension. I applaud the attention being paid to this important connection, which has so long been ignored. I again want to caution that many of the recommendations still belong in the experimental category, and it will be many years before the final recommendations can be made. I have concerns for significant imbalancing of the normal amino acid patterns found in healthful food. There seems to be no question that increasing quantities of lysine help to protect against virus infections, including herpes, chicken pox, and shingles, and there is some less substantive evidence that it is protective against certain malignancies that may possibly be related to such virus infections. However, the prolonged imbalance produced by such excessive intake of lysine with respect to arginine can have theoretically significant long-term effects which may not be the optimal way to go for all people. Increasing the intake of arginine to balance the lysine negates the efficacy of the lysine therapy. Some Life Extension proponents recommend high intakes of arginine, and this could tend to increase susceptibility to the viruses. Obviously, the ultimate answer is not available.

Similarly, we can manipulate amino acids to produce mood changes. Amino acids such as serotonin, norepinephrine, dopamine, and so on, help the central nervous system communicate from one nerve cell to another. Not only do they produce new changes but they also alter sleep patterns, appetite, appreciation of pain, and other manifestations of proper function of the brain and peripheral nervous system. In some situations, they can obviate the need for drugs and in my opinion are clearly preferable to pharmacological agents which are foreign to the body's metabolic machinery.

Examples are drugs used for tranquilizers, antidepressants, mood elevaters, appetite suppressants, hypnotics, and sedatives. However, as is certainly true with these classes of drugs, the long-term use of even natural substances which affect behavior should be under the guidance of a physician knowledgeable in this form of therapeutic nutrition.

The final category of supplementation is in the area of minerals and should include the following:

Calcium	1000 mg
Magnesium	1000 mg
Zinc	15 mg
Iron	15 mg
Manganese	10 mg
Copper	1 mg
Chromium	200 mcg
Iodine	150 mcg

It is my opinion that the best absorbed form of these minerals is not as a salt of common mineral acids, such as chlorides and sulfates, nor as the oxide, hydroxide, or carbonate forms, but rather as complexes with amino acids (chelated), or weak organic acids such as aspartate, orotate, or lactate. The doses specified are for the elemental amounts. For instance, 500 milligrams of calcium orotate contain approximately 100 milligrams of elemental calcium. Most supplements include that information on the label.

Other mineral substances are sometimes recommended, including phosphorous, molybdenum, germanium, rubidium, vanadium, nickel, and so on. The evidence for the importance of minute quantities of these substances is certainly strong, but to date the appropriate amounts are still a mystery, according to most authorities. There is a significant possibility that in the attempt to supplement with these factors, excess quantities could build up and evidence for toxicity is almost as strong as for the requirement. These substances are among those that are best obtained from quality foods carefully grown in healthy soil.

—Warren M. Levin, M.D.

Drug Induced Nutritional Deficiencies

We have established that the immune system is compromised in the presence of malnutrition. Drug-induced nutritional deficiencies—

particularly vitamin deficiencies—are among the ten leading causes of malnutrition in America today. Robert J. Benowicz, biochemist and author of *Vitamins and You* and *Non-Prescription Drugs and their Side Effects,* shares this information for *In Pursuit of Youth:*

THE MUSHROOMING PHENOMENON

The widespread and frequent use of medications, whether by prescription, over-the-counter, or recreational, is a mushrooming phenomenon. Unfortunately, most drugs are powerful chemical agents as alien to human tissues and metabolism as the noxious and toxic pollutants of our contemporary environment. The body recognizes the vast majority as poisonous and responds with biochemical mechanisms to neutralize and eliminate these foreign substance(s) as rapidly as possible. Such detoxification relies on enzymatic breakdown of the pharmaceutical compound(s), whose presence increases your dietary need for vitamin co-enzymes. This elevated demand for additional nutrients raises your personal need for specific vitamins and can produce outright or clinical malnutrition if your diet fails to provide increased quantities of the necessary co-enzymes. It is a dietary burden, or stress factor, that lasts as long as you continue to take a medication. For example, if you take aspirin on a daily basis for the relief of arthritis pain and inflammation, you automatically increase your personal requirement for ☆**vitamin C**☆ for as long as you continue to take this analgesic.

With an increasing tendency, particularly among senior citizens, to take one or more medication(s) on a daily basis, often for months or years at a time, it is important to know what additional demands are being made by the drugs you use so that dietary compensation can be made through foods or vitamin supplements. Indeed, it is a wise rule of thumb not to accept any prescription for long-term medication without closely questioning your physician about its potential for damaging your nutritional well-being and the wisdom of taking nutritional supplements to compensate for the kinds of damage that potentially accompany your drug therapy.

Be particularly aware that:

• Antibiotics, e.g., neomycin, tetracycline, penicillin, etc., interfere with the absorption of fat-soluble vitamins (A and K) from the digestive tract into the circulatory system. Additional quantities of these vitamins may be necessary during drug therapy.

- Regular laxative use, particularly of mineral oil, interferes with the absorption of fat-soluble vitamins (A, D, E, and K) from the digestive tract. If you use mineral oil on a regular basis, be certain you are getting adequate quantities of these nutrients.
- Prolonged use of cholesterol lowering drugs, e.g., Questran, interferes with the absorption of fat-soluble vitamins A and D and water-soluble B_{12} from the gut. Consult your physician about the advisability of supplementation.
- Diabetics and people with hyperthyroid metabolism have difficulty in converting beta carotene (provitamin A from plant sources) into usable vitamin A and may require supplementation with the preformed vitamin, particularly if they are being treated with insulin, oral hypoglycemics, or thyroid medications.
- Anticonvulsant medications, e.g., Dilantin, phenobarbital, phosphate-containing laxatives, and sleep-inducing drugs containing glutethimide, e.g., Doriden, increase your need for vitamin D if such drugs are taken on a regular basis.
- The mineral iron, and various thyroid hormones are biochemical antagonists of vitamin E. Their regular use will increase your need for the nutrient. In contrast, E may enhance the blood-thinning effects of anticoagulants, e.g., Coumadin, more than therapeutically intended and lead to internal hemorrhaging. Consult your physician about the simultaneous use of such drugs and the vitamin.
- Over-the-counter antacids tend to deplete the body's supplies of all water-soluble vitamins (C, B_1, B_2, B_3, B_6, B_{12}, folic acid, biotin, cholines, and pantothenic acid). Regular antacid use requires additional intake of these nutrients.
- Diuretics accelerate the flushing of water-soluble vitamins and minerals from the body. Frequent use of such dehydrating drugs, e.g., diuretics, "water pills," antihypertensives, etc., raises your dietary requirement for C, B_1, B_2, B_3, B_{12}, folic acid, and biotin. Biotin, in particular, may be an important nutritional adjunct to prolonged drug therapy.
- The frequent use of prescription analgesics, e.g., Indocin; or over-the-counter products, e.g., aspirin or other salicylate; anticoagulants, e.g., Coumadin; antidepressants, e.g., Permitil; and steroids, e.g., Cortisone, tend to increase the body's demand for vi-

tamin C, and supplementation with the vitamin is probably advisable during therapy.

- Ascorbic acid (the usual form of vitamin C) makes urine more acidic, and in the presence of sulfa drugs, e.g., Gantrisin, may upset kidney chemistry. Use of ascorbate forms of the vitamin avoids this problem, but be certain to inform your physician of supplementation with C before taking any sulfa medication.

- Riboflavin (B_2) and folic acid are significant factors in the detoxification of methotrexate used in chemotherapy. Achieving a proper balance between these vitamins and the drug is critical to avoid nutritional deficiencies without reducing therapeutic effectiveness of the medication. Consult your physician.

- Daily use of antidepressants, e.g., Elavil; estrogens, e.g., Premarin; hydralazine-containing antihypertensives, e.g., Apresoline; isoniazid-containing drugs for the treatment of tuberculosis, e.g., Rifamate; and penicillamine-containing drugs for the treatment of arthritis all tend to increase the body's requirements for vitamin B_6. Consult your physician.

- Antigout medications containing colchinine, e.g., Colbenemid; anticoagulant drugs, e.g., Coumadin; and potassium supplements, e.g., Kaochlor (used to compensate for the loss of potassium during diuretic/antihypertensive drug therapy) tend to block absorption of vitamin B_{12} from the digestive tract. Supplementation with the vitamin may be wise. Consult your physician.

—Robert J. Benowicz

The Greasy Spoon

The very word "fat" is a turn-off. "Fathead" or "fat chance" have unpleasant associations. "Greasy spoon" conjures up negative images, as does "blubber" or "tub of lard." Yet fatty acids are found in every tissue cell of your body.

We are getting many messages: too much fat is no good; the right kind of fat is important; the transformation of fat in metabolism is even more significant; the ratio of one fat to another is crucial; rancidity of fat is harmful; the Eskimos eat polyunsaturated fat (look how healthy they are); the Masai consume animal fat (look how healthy they are). Do you have to have a Ph.D. in biochemistry to understand it all? Possibly. But there are a few facts that should be part of your armamentarium in your pursuit for youth.

- Essential fatty acids play a role in emotional disorders. People under emotional stress have depressed immune systems. It is theorized that because essential fatty acids promote T-lymphocyte activity, this immune system booster has a positive effect on emotions.[18]
- Abnormal proportions of polyunsaturated and saturated fats are found in women with breast cancer. Partial correction is accomplished with gamma linolenic acid (GLA) supplementation. This kind of supplementation has also been reported to alleviate breast tenderness. In one study, six grams of GLA daily was administered to women with fibrocystic disease, with positive results.[19]
- Inadequate intake of essential fatty acids may also explain why changes in ear wax composition are related to certain aspects of malignancy risk: when ear wax becomes very hard and does not soften at body temperature, it may indicate a much higher proportion of certain fatty acids that have not metabolized properly.[20]
- GLA is a precursor of prostaglandin E_1: GLA is necessary for the manufacture of prostaglandins which in turn activate T-lymphocytes, and inhibit smooth muscle proliferation and thrombosis, among other attributes. GLA can only be manufactured in the body through a complex series of metabolic processes. This function declines with age; is impaired in experimental manipulation which accelerates aging; and is enhanced in those situations known to be associated with delayed aging.

GLA administration has been found to lower blood pressure and cholesterol, and to cause clinical improvement in patients with scleroderma and alcoholism. These diseases are associated with some features of accelerated aging. The mechanism at work is a blocked enzyme, which can be by-passed by giving GLA directly.[21]

- The chemical malonaldehyde forms when polyunsaturated fats are broken down by air. It is present in large amounts in many common foods, ranging from beef to peanut butter. Dr. Raymond Shamberger, a Cleveland biochemist, found that six milligrams of malonaldehyde applied to the skin of a mouse produces cancer. It is Dr. Shamberger's contention that seventy-five grams of this chemical consumed in a lifetime may be a key factor in causing cancer of the gastrointestinal tract.

Beef is the food with the highest level of malonaldehyde. A sirloin tip roast, uncooked, contains 9.4 milligrams of malonaldehyde per gram of meat. When roasted, the level jumps to 27 milligrams per gram. A freshly opened jar of peanut butter contains no malonaldehyde, but after it has been opened and used for some time, it contains 1.2 milligrams per gram.

Refrigeration, vitamins C and E, and the mineral selenium reduce the carcinogenic effects of malonaldehyde. Raw vegetables, high in vitamin C, are the best antidote.

- Excellent sources of polyunsaturated fats are contained in fresh, natural foods: avocados, sunflower seeds, nuts, cold water fish, mammalian organ tissues (liver). Added insurance? Gamma linolenic supplementation.

Bottom of the Totem Pole

We're not doing so well in America. The American female ranks only eleventh in the world in life expectancy. In the 20-year-old age group, American females will be outlived by 20-year-old females in twenty-one other countries. American males in that same age group will be outlived by males in thirty-six countries. Males in the 41-year-old age group have only a 4.1 year longer life expectancy compared to seventy-six years ago, despite all the modern medical achievements of the past century.

On the scale of life expectancy, we rank twenty-first, with a 66.6-year life expectancy, and eighteenth in the number of infant deaths under one year of age per thousand live births. (That means it's safer to have a baby in seventeen other countries!)[22]

WHAT ABOUT KEITH?

There are two kinds of hospital patients: those who complain about the hospital food, and those who are on intravenous feeding. Keith is not well enough to complain just yet, but he is wondering why it happened.

Evidence is mounting that exercise may increase the liability to heart disease in particular cases. If untrained, the jogger may develop an occlusion (closing) of a coronary vessel. Hardening of coronary vessels prevents a normal response to the oxygen demands of exercise. The increase of blood flow may dislodge a thrombus from the arterial wall and this can then block a smaller vessel. Platelet aggregation is increased following maximum stress, which may cause partial occlusion of an artery to become complete.

It is difficult to identify the individual who will respond unfavorably. Possible clues are an aggressive, competitive personality, with reluctance to accept the slow progression of exercise necessary for a safe program.[23]

The question is not whether to exercise, but when to do it and to what extent, and how to consume nutrients that contribute to heart health. Harmful effects of very strenuous efforts are often associated with great emotional strain (fear and/or anxiety). At such times the physical effort is overpowered by an acute catecholamine storm (the sympathetic system's hormone release), by exhaustion, by circulatory collapse, and signs of acute myocardial ischemia. Dr. Z. Fejfar of the Cardiovascular Research Center in Czechoslovakia says:

The simple equation, energy balance equals energy expenditure and dietary intake, becomes a rather complicated matter in a life situation, where many factors—age, environmental changes, and disease—may interact or intervene. . . . Adaptation must be at the level of the heart muscle cell, in the mitochondrial enzyme structure and function.[24]

We have discussed elements and processes which promote health on a cellular level, thereby supporting the immune system. They are the same ingredients which promote youth.

There are so many components of the immune response, and many aspects for study. The information is emerging so fast that it is difficult to totally absorb it. In the excitement of technological research, we must not forget that we've been around a long time. It's thrilling to understand highly detailed and complex mechanisms at work through advanced space age procedures. But we don't necessarily require that knowledge in our personal pursuit of youth. The answer has been around a long time. Hippocrates knew it. He said: "Healing is a matter of time, but it is sometimes also a matter of opportunity."

Flying Hawk knew it too. In the 1800s he said: "Indians and animals know better how to live than white man; nobody can be in good health if he does not have all the time good food, fresh air, sunshine, and good water."

APPENDIX

RESOURCES

Cookbooks

Frank Ford, *The Simpler Life Cookbook* (Fort Worth, TX: Harvest Press, 1974).

Marjorie Winn Ford, Susan Hillyard, and Mary Faulk Koock, *The Deaf Smith Country Cookbook* (New York: Collier Books, 1973).

Betty Kamen and Si Kamen, *The Kamen Plan for Total Nutrition During Pregnancy* (Norwalk, CT: Appleton-Century-Crofts, 1981). Over 100 pages of food and recipe information.

Betty Kamen and Si Kamen, *Kids Are What They Eat: What Every Parent Needs to Know About Nutrition* (New York: Arco Publishing, Inc., 1983). Recipe section.

Ken Neumeyer, *Sailing the Farm* (Berkeley, CA: Ten-Speed Press, 1982).

Magazines

Health Facts, 237 Thompson St., New York, NY 10012.

Let's Live, 444 N. Larchmont Blvd., Los Angeles, CA 90004.

Your Good Health, Keats Publishing Co., 27 Pine St., New Canaan, CT 06840.

Books for Pregnancy and Parenting

Betty Kamen and Si Kamen, *The Kamen Plan for Total Nutrition During Pregnancy* (Norwalk, CT: Appleton-Century-Crofts, 1981).

Betty Kamen and Si Kamen, *Kids Are What They Eat: What Every Parent Needs to Know About Nutrition* (New York: Arco Publishing, Inc., 1983).

Organizations

Center for Medical Consumers and Health Care Information, Inc., 237 Thompson St., New York, NY 10012.

Huxley Institute, 219 East 31st St., New York, NY 10016.

International Academy of Preventive Medicine, Suite 469, 34 Corporate Woods, Overland Park, KA 66210.

National Health Federation, 212 Foothill Blvd, Monrovia, CA 91016.

Filmstrips for Nutrition Education

Encore Visual Education, Inc., 1235 South Victory Blvd., Burbank, CA 91502; (213) 843-6515:

> *Beans, Beans, Beans*
> *Fruitful Menu*
> *Grain Cookery*
> *Vegetarianism: Healthful Eating*
> *Food: The Choice Is Yours*
> *The Tofu Experience*
> *Kitchen With a Mission: Nutrition*
> *The Seed Sprout Secret*
> *The Peanut Butter Caper*

Bergwall Productions, 839 Stewart Ave., P.O. Box 238, Garden City, NY 11520; (800) 645-3565.

> Exploding Nutrition Myths-1
> > *The Food-Group Foolers*
> > *The Protein Picture*
> > *The Grain Robbery*
> > *The Milky Way*
> > *Give Produce Priority*
> > *Striking oil*
> Exploding Nutrition Myths-2
> > *Dietary Goals*
> > *The Sad State of Overweight*
> > *Complex Carbohydrates Simplified*
> > *Sugar: Not Such Sweet Talk*
> > *Cut the Fat*
> > *The Salt Shake-Up*
> > *Beyond the New Health Horizon*

HOW TO SPROUT

Sprouting Equipment

The best equipment for sprouting is the one-quart canning jar. These jars are widemouthed, withstand boiling water for thorough cleansing, and are quite durable. They range in cost from one to three dollars each, depending on whether you are shopping in John's bargain basement or Bloomingdale's. Discard the glass tops, rubber rings, and metal wires. All you need is the jar.

Buy nylon mosquito netting at a hardware store, and dig out some short, thick rubber bands. (You must have some in that "catch-all" drawer in the kitchen.) Cut the netting into squares large enough to cover the tops of the jars, and secure with the rubber bands. This is the best and cheapest sprouting equipment available.

Sprouting Instructions

Soak each variety of seeds or beans in one cup of water in a jar overnight. It is preferable to use pure spring water for the soaking procedure. Recommended quantities:

alfalfa	one tablespoon
mung	two tablespoons
radish	one-half tablespoon
azuki	two tablespoons
chick-peas	three tablespoons
lentils	two tablespoons
sunflower seeds	two tablespoons
soybeans	one tablespoon
wheatberries	two tablespoons
buckwheat	two tablespoons
clover	one tablespoon
rye	one tablespoon
sesame	one tablespoon

In the morning, pour the water off. (Use this water for your plants—they'll love it! Or save the water to use as stock.) Dumping the seeds into a strainer facilitates the washing process. Rinse thoroughly under the faucet.

Return seeds to jar after shaking strainer by tapping against side of sink. Cover jar with nylon mesh netting and tight rubber band.

Place jar upside down at slight angle in dish rack, so that remaining water can run off. Sprouts appreciate moisture, but not puddles. Rinse seeds again in the evening. If you can rinse again in the middle of the day, that's an advantage. Now that the seeds are no longer soaking in water, they can be rinsed directly under faucet in the jars. The mesh netting, held in place with the rubber band, prevents the seeds from escaping when the water is poured off. (Be sure the rubber band is tight enough.)

Many people start the procedure in the dark because this expedites growth. We, however, find that when we hide the jars in a closet, we forget about them. When we unveil them a week or so later, it is not unlike Pandora's box. Another possibility is to place the jar in a paper bag and leave it on the kitchen counter as a reminder. We don't bother with this procedure either since sprouts that have germinated in daylight develop with more nutrients.

Seeds may be consumed at any stage of sprouting, but harvesting at peak offers the most value. Vitamin C is actually synthesized during germination, and the concentrations of some of the B vitamins is also increased, along with other nutrients.

The peak germination time for the most popular seeds is: alfalfa, 4 days; mung, 3 days; radish, 4 days; azuki, 2 days; chick-peas, 1 day; lentils, 2 days; sunflower seeds, 1 day; soybeans, 1 or 2 days; wheatberries, 2 or 3 days; buckwheat, 3 or 4 days; clover, 4 days; rye, 2 days; sesame, 1 or 2 days.

Since seeds vary, it is advisable to experiment, using a good sprouting book as a guide. Alfalfa, mung, and chick-peas are excellent sprouts for beginners. Before consuming, leave sprouts in indirect sunlight. This will "green" the leaves, adding chlorophyll.

Refrigerated sprouts will last up to a week. But since they are growing in your kitchen, the "farm" couldn't be any closer. It is best to "harvest" as needed to optimize nutrient value. Sprouts are so inexpensive that you may discard, rather than save any surplus. (For the novice: "harvesting sprouts" simply means taking them from the jar.)

REFERENCES

Chapter 1: The Exercise Connection

1. Jeffrey Bland, Symposium: Nutritional Approaches to the Management of Intestinal Disorders, Autoimmune Phenomena, and Endocrinopathies, New York City, March 19 & 20, 1983.
2. Jeffrey P. Koplan et al., "An Epidemiologic Study of the Benefits and Risks of Running," *Journal of the American Medical Association* 248 (December 1982):3118.

3. Thomas G. Pickering, "Runner's Radial Palsy," *New England Journal of Medicine* 305 (September 24, 1981):768.

4. Lee M. Jampol and Jay A. Fleischman, "Central Retinal-Vein Occlusion Five Days After a Marathon," *New England Journal of Medicine* 305 (September 24, 1981):764.

5. Fred Levit, "Joggers Nipples," *New England Journal of Medicine* 297 (1977):1127.

6. P. Siltanen and M. Kekki, "Effect of Exercise on the Formed Elements of Urinary Sediment," *Acta Medica Scandinavica* 164 (1959):151–157.

7. J. Widdicombe, "Respiratory Reflexes," in *Handbook of Physiology: Respiration,* Section 3, vol. 1, eds. W. Fenn and H. Rahn (Washington, D.C.: American Physiological Society, 1964), pp. 585–630.

8. T. Kavanagh, "A Cold-weather 'Jogging Mask' for Angina Patients," *Canadian Medical Association Journal* 103 (1970):1290–91.

9. Sharon H. Vitousek, "Is More Better?" *Nutrition Today* 14 (November–December 1979):10–17.

10. Colm O'Herlihy, "Jogging and Suppression of Ovulation," *New England Journal of Medicine* 306 (January 7, 1982):50.

11. A. B. Corrigan and K. D. Fitch, "Complications of Jogging," *Medical Journal of Australia* 2 (August 12, 1972):363–68.

12. Don Mannerberg and June Roth, *Aerobic Nutrition* (New York: Hawthorn/Dutton, 1981), p. 62.

13. Corrigan and Fitch, *op. cit.*

14. Melvin Hershkowitz, "Penile Frostbite, An Unforeseen Hazard of Jogging," *New England Journal of Medicine* vol. 296 (January 20, 1977):178.

15. Raymond Dreyfack, *The Complete Book of Walking* (Rockville Centre, New York: Farnsworth Publishing Co., Inc., 1979), pp. 189–204.

16. Editorial, "Blood and Sports," *Lancet* 2 (October 17, 1981):847–48.

17. *Ibid.*

18. John H. Kleinman, "Brachial Plexus Injury from Tight Backpack Straps," *New England Journal of Medicine* 305 (August 27, 1981):524–25.

19. Dreyfack, *op. cit.*

20. Drummond Rennie and Norman K. Hollenberg, "Cardiomythology and Marathons," *New England Journal of Medicine* 301 (July 12, 1979):103–4.

21. Beat Steinman, Richard Gitzelmann, and Milo Zachmann, "Catecholamines, Dopamine, and Endorphin Levels During Extreme Exercise," *New England Journal of Medicine* 305 (August 20, 1981):466–67.

22. John M. Douglass and Sue Douglass, "Light," *Your Health,* newsletter of the International Academy of Preventive Medicine (July 1983):1.

23. J. P. Nicholson and D. B. Case, "Carboxyhemoglobin Levels in New York Runners," *Physician and Sports Medicine* 2 (March 1983):137.

24. Alan M. Smith, "Butter," *Lancet* 1 (April 23, 1983):929–30.

25. Jeffrey Bland, *Your Health Under Siege: Using Nutrition to Fight Back* (Brattleboro, Vermont: The Stephen Greene Press, 1981), p. 90.

26. Saul Kent, *The Life Extension Revolution: The Definitive Guide to Better Health, Longer Life, and Physical Immortality* (New York : William Morrow and Co., Inc., 1980), p. 168.

27. Gary E. Gibson and Christine Peterson, "Biochemical and Behavioral Parallels in Aging and Hypoxia," in *The Aging Brain: Cellular and Molecular Mechanisms of Aging in the Nervous System*, vol. 20, eds. Ezio Giacobini et al. (New York: Raven Press, 1982), pp. 107, 119.

28. Fitzgerald W. Labile, "Hypertension and Jogging: New Diagnostic Tool or Spurious Discovery?" *British Medical Journal* 282 (1981):542–44.

29. Interview with Raymond Dreyfack, WMCA Radio, New York, September 1979.

30. Rennie and Hollenberg, *op. cit.*

31. Waneen Wyrick Spirduso, "Physical Fitness in Relation to Motor Aging," *The Aging Motor System: Advances in Neurogerontology*, vol. 3, eds. Francis J. Pirozzolo and Gabe J. Maletta (New York: Praeger Publishers, 1982), p. 121.

32. *Ibid.*

33. *Ibid.*

34. J. S. Skinner, "The Cardiovascular System with Aging and Exercise," in *Medicine and Sport: Physical Activity and Aging*, vol. 4, eds. D. Brunner and E. Jokl (Basel: Karger, 1970), pp. 100–108.

35. S. P. Tzankoff et al., "Physiological Adjustments to Work in Older Men as Affected by Physical Training," *Journal of Applied Physiology* 33 (1972):346–50.

36. B. A. Stamford, "Effects of Chronic Institutionalization on the Physical Working Capacity and Trainability of Geriatric Men," *Journal of Gerontology* 28 (1973):441–46.

37. H. A. deVries, "Physiology of Exercise and Aging," in *Physical Activity and Human Well-Being*, eds. F. Landry and W.A.R. Orban (Miami: Symposia Specialists, 1978), p. 516.

38. W. W. Spirduso, "Physical Fitness, Aging, and Psychomotor Speed: A Review," *Journal of Gerontology* 35 (1980):850–65.

39. Lawrence E. Lamb, "Exercise, Posture, Strength," *The Health Letter* 1 (1973):1–4.

40. "New Research Findings on Walking: Nature's Own Amazing 'Anti-Age Antibiotic,' " *Executive Health* 14 (July 1978):1–4.

41. *Ibid.*, p. 1.

42. Spirduso, *op. cit.*

43. A. G. Frantz and M. T. Rabkin, "Effects of Estrogen and Sex Differences on Secretion of Human Growth Hormone," *Journal of Clinical Endocrinology and Metabolism* 25 (1965):1470–80.

44. W. M. Hunter, C. C. Fonseka, and R. Passmore, "The Role of Growth Hormone in the Mobilization of Fuel for Muscular Exercise," *Quarterly Journal of Experimental Physiology* 50 (1965):406–16.

45. *Executive Health*, *op. cit.*, p. 2.

46. *Ibid.*

47. Myron Winick, "Introduction," in *Killer Diseases*, ed. Myron Winick (New York: John Wiley and Sons, 1981), p. 12.

48. Philip Felig et al., "Hypoglycemia During Prolonged Exercise in Normal Men," *New England Journal of Medicine* 306 (April 15, 1982):895–900.

49. Vitousek, *op. cit.*

50. J. D. Brooke, "Carbohydrate Nutrition and Human Performance," in *Nutrition, Physical Fitness, and Health*, International Series on Sport Sciences, vol. 7, eds. Jana Parizkova and V.A. Rogozkin (Baltimore: University Park Press, 1978), pp. 42–52.

51. J. Parizkova, "Body Composition and Lipid Metabolism in Relation to Nutrition and Exercise," in *Nutrition, Physical Fitness, and Health*, International Series on Sport Sciences, vol. 7, eds. Jana Parizkova and V. A. Rogozkin (Baltimore: University Park Press, 1978), pp. 61–75.

52. D. L. Costill et al., "The Role of Dietary Carbohydrates in Muscle Glycogen Resynthesis After Strenuous Running," *American Journal of Clinical Nutrition* 34 (September 1981):1831–36.

53. K. Bergström et al., "Diet, Muscle Glycogen and Physical Performance," *Acta Physiologica Scandinavica* 71 (1967):140.

54. Vitousek, *op. cit.*

55. G. H. Hartung, William G. Squires, and Antonio M. Gotto, "Effect of Exercise Training on Plasma High-Density Lipoprotein Cholesterol in Coronary Disease Patients," *American Heart Journal* 101 (1981):181–84.

56. Roy J. Shephard, *Physiology and Biochemistry of Exercise* (New York: Praeger Publishers, 1982), pp. 37–40.

57. Daniel F. Hanley, "Athletic Training and How Diet Affects It," *Nutrition Today* 14 (November–December 1979):5–9.

58. W. S. S. Ladell and R. A. Kenney, "Some Laboratory and Field Observations on the Harvard Pack Test," *Quarterly Journal of Experimental Physiology* 40 (1955):283–96.

59. Leif Hallberg and Lena Rossander, "Absorption of Iron from Western-Type Lunch and Dinner Meals," *American Journal of Clinical Nutrition* 35 (March 1982):502–9.

60. N. G. Norgan and A. Ferro-Luzzi, "Nutrition, Physical Activity and Physical Fitness in Contrasting Environments," in *Nutrition, Physical Fitness, and Health*, eds. Jana Parizkova and V. A. Rogozkin (Baltimore: University Park Press, 1978), p. 185.

61. M. J. Karvonen, "Nutrition in Heavy Manual Labor," in *Nutrition and Physical Activity*, V *Symposium of Swedish Nutrition Foundation* (Uppsala: G. Blix, 1967), pp. 59–63.

62. "FAO/WHO Requirements of Vitamin A, Thiamine, Riboflavin and Niacin," *World Health Organization Technical Report Series* (1967):1–86.

63. Shephard, *op. cit.*, pp. 40–41.

64. N. B. Strydom et al., "Changes in the Level of Serum Vitamin C in Mineworkers," *Journal of South African Institute Mining Metals,* 77 (1977):214–17.
65. R. E. Johnson et al., "Effects of Variations in Dietary Vitamin C on the Physical Well-Being of Manual Workers," *Journal of Nutrition* 29 (1945):155–65.
66. D. H. Horstman, "Nutrition," in *Ergogenic Aids and Muscular Performance,* ed. W. P. Morgan (New York: Academic Press, 1972), pp. 343–65.
67. A. Hoogerweref and A. W. J. H. Hoitink, "The Influence of Vitamin C Administration on the Mechanical Efficiency of the Human Organism," *Physiology* 20 (1963):164–72.
68. W. D. Van Huss, "What Makes the Russians Run?" *Nutrition Today* 1 (1966):20–23.
69. Roy J. Shepard et al., "Vitamin E, Exercise and the Recovery from Physical Activity," *Journal of Applied Physiology* 333 (1974):119–26.
70. Y. Kobayashi, "Effect of Vitamin E on Aerobic Work Performance in Man During Acute Exposure to Hypoxic Hypoxial," Ph.D. Thesis, University of New Mexico, Albuquerque, New Mexico, 1974.
71. Mannerberg and Roth, *op cit.,* p. 37.
72. Helen E. Fisher, Ph.D., anthropologist with the New York Academy of Sciences, personal letter, May 1983. Personal Files of Betty and Si Kamen, Larkspur, CA.
73. Robert E. Olson, "Energy Requirements: How Much is Enough?" *Nutrition Reviews* 40 (May 5, 1982):160.
74. "Exercise, Health and Medicine," Symposium, *Lancet* 1 (May 21, 1983):1171.
75. Lamb, *op. cit.*
76. *Ibid.*
77. Richard A. Kunin, *Mega-Nutrition: The New Prescription for Maximum Health, Energy and Longevity* (New York: McGraw-Hill Book Co., 1980), p. 174.
78. Marian Thompson Arlin, *The Science of Nutrition* (New York: Macmillan Publishing Co., 1972), p. 87.
79. N. Hickey et al., "Study of Coronary Risk Factors Related to Physical Activity in 15,171 Men," *British Medical Journal* 30 (August 1975):507–9.
80. S. Suzuki and S. Oshima, "Influence of Physical Exercise on Blood Pressure Using the Spontaneously Hypertensive Rat," *Japanese Journal of Nutrition* 34 (1976):109–14.
81. Mannerberg and Roth, *op. cit.,* p. 37.
82. Michael Kamen, M.A., education consultant, personal letter, July 1983. Personal Files of Betty and Si Kamen, Larkspur, CA.

83. M. S. Pollock et al., "Effects of Mode of Training on Cardiovascular Function and Body Composition of Adult Men," *Medical Science of Sports* 7 (1975):139–45.

84. J. E. Carter and W. H. Phillips, "Structural Changes in Exercising Middle-Aged Males During a Two-Year Period," *Journal of Applied Physiology* 27 (1969):787–94.

85. K. H. Sidney, R. J. Shepard, and J. Harrison, "Endurance Training and Body Composition of the Elderly," *American Journal of Clinical Nutrition* 30 (1977):326–33.

86. Kenneth Cooper, *Your Health: Journal of the International Academy of Preventive Medicine* (July 1983):2.

87. "Warming Up and Cooling Down," in *The Health and Fitness Handbook*, ed. Miriam Polunin (New York: Van Nostrand Reinhold Co., 1981), p. 69.

88. Ned Bayrd and Chris Quilter, *Food For Champions: How to Eat to Win* (Boston: Houghton Mifflin Co., 1982), p. 78.

89. M. B. Jorksten and B. Jonsson, "Endurance Limit of Force in Long Term Intermittent Static Contractions," *Work and Environmental Health* 3 (1977):23–27.

90. "How the Body Reacts to Stress," in *The Health and Fitness Handbook*, op. cit., p. 176.

91. Alayne Yates, Kevin Leehey, and Catherine M. Shisslak, "Running: An Analogue of Anorexia?" *New England Journal of Medicine* 308 (February 3, 1983):251–55.

92. "Exercise, Health, and Medicine," Symposium, *Lancet* 1 (May 21, 1983):1171.

93. *New York Post*, July 19, 1983, "Workers Told Exercise Is Hazardous to Health."

Chapter 2: Image Projection

1. Arthur Stringer, "A Fragile Thing Is Beauty," stanza 2, in *Bartlett's Familiar Quotations*, centennial edition, ed. John Bartlett (Boston: Little, Brown and Co., 1955), p. 878a.

2. Mark E. Williams and Norin M. Hadler, "Sounding Board: The Illness as the Focus of Geriatric Medicine," *New England Journal of Medicine* 308 (June 2, 1983):1357–60.

3. Gilbert Martin-Bouyer, "Outbreak of Accidental Hexachlorophene Poisoning in France," *Lancet* 1 (January 9, 1982):91–95.

4. R. W. Anderson et al., "Risk of Handling Injectable Antineoplastic Agents," *American Journal of Hospital Pharmacology* 39 (1982):1881–87.

5. Maurice Hirst et al., "Caution On Handling Antineoplastic Drugs," *New England Journal of Medicine* 309 (July 21, 1983):188–89.

6. Randi J. Hagerman and Andrew Levitas, "Dilantin and the Fragile X Syndrome," *New England Journal of Medicine* 308 (June 9, 1983):1424.
7. Joe Graedon, *The People's Pharmacy* 2 (New York: Avon Books, 1980), p. 201.
8. L. Ovesen, "Drugs and Vitamin Deficiency," *Drugs* 18 (1979):278–98.
9. Eric Wilkes, *Drug Management of Chronic Disease and Other Problems* (London: Faber and Faber, 1982), p. 269.
10. Harry W. Daniell, "A Study in the Epidemiology of Crow's Feet," *Annals of Internal Medicine* 75 (1971):873–80.
11. Frederic Speer, *Food Allergy* (Littleton, MA: PSG Publishing Co., Inc., 1979), p. 32.
12. Marta Fiorotto and Buford L. Nichols, "Edema of Malnutrition," *Lancet* 2 (October 16, 1982):871.
13. Richard A. Kunin, *Mega-Nutrition for Women* (New York: McGraw-Hill Book Co., 1983), p. 54.
14. Carl C. Pfeiffer, *Mental and Elemental Nutrients: A Physician's Guide to Nutrition and Health Care* (New Canaan, CT: Keats Publishing Co., 1975), p. 183.
15. Dr. John M. Douglass and Sue Douglass, "Light," *Your Health*, International Academy of Preventive Medicine Newsletter (July 1983):1.
16. Roger J. Williams, *Physician's Handbook of Nutritional Science* (Springfield, IL: Charles C. Thomas Publishers, 1975), p. 6.
17. Jeffrey Bland, Symposium: Nutritional Approaches to the Management of Intestinal Disorders, Autoimmune Phenomena, and Endocrinopathies, New York City, March 19 & 20, 1983.
18. Emil Ginter, "Ascorbic Acid in Cholesterol and Bile Acid Metabolism," *Annals of the New York Academy of Sciences* 258 (1975):410–21.
19. *Ibid.*
20. David A. Fenton and John D. Wilkinson, "Dose-Related Visual-Field Defects in Patients Receiving PUVA Therapy," *Lancet* 1 (May 14, 1983):1106.
21. John M. Douglass, "Psoriasis and Diet," *The Western Journal of Medicine* 133 (November 1980):450.
22. David Stoll and Lloyd E. King, "Disulfiram-Alcohol Skin Reaction to Beer-Containing Shampoo," *Journal of the American Medical Association* 244 (November 7, 1980):2045.
23. Allan Astrup Jensen, "Melanoma, Fluorescent Lights, and Polychlorinated Biphenyls," *Lancet* 2 (October 23, 1982):935.
24. "Malignant Melanoma and Exposure to Fluorescent Lighting at Work Confirmed," *International Journal of Biosocial Research* 4 (1983):99.
25. Lance R. Peterson, LoAnn C. Peterson, and Anja K. Peterson, "French Vanilla Frostbite," *New England Journal of Medicine* 307 (October 14, 1982):1028.

26. Harvey J. Cohen, "Joggers' Petechiae," *New England Journal of Medicine* 279 (July 11, 1968):109.
27. Grant R. Gwinup, "The Sunglass Syndrome," *New England Journal of Medicine* 309 (May 12, 1983):1168.
28. Chin Shih, "Mishaps of CPR: The Case of the Missing Dental Bridge," *New England Journal of Medicine* 306 (April 29, 1982):1057.
29. William Shakespeare, *Henry IV, Second Part*, I.ii, in *Dictionary of Quotations*, ed. Bergen Evans (New York: Avenel Books, 1978), p. 11.
30. Arieh Bergman et al., "Acceleration of Wound Healing by Topical Application of Honey," *American Journal of Surgery* 145 (March 1983):374.
31. Jorge Chirife and León Herszage, "Sugar for Infected Wounds," *Lancet* 2 (July 17, 1982):157.
32. B. Rose, "Honey or Sugar in Treatment of Infected Wounds?" *Lancet* 1 (April 24, 1982):963.
33. Renate Lewin, "Aloe Vera: Rediscovering the Healing Desert Lily," *Health Quarterly* (May–June 1982):12,58.
34. "Gold Trading Table," *Washington Post*, (August 14, 1982):D10.
35. James F. Burris, "Drugs Worth More Than Their Weight in Gold," letter to *New England Journal of Medicine* 307 (November 18, 1982):1350.
36. Samuel D. McFadden, "Drugs Worth More Than Their Weight in Gold," letter to *New England Journal of Medicine* 308 (March 31, 1983):783.
37. Russell Colber, "Drugs Worth More Than Their Weight in Gold," letter to *New England Journal of Medicine* 308 (March 31, 1983):783.
38. Jeanne Rose, *Herbal Body Book* (New York: Grosset and Dunlap, 1976), p. 105.
39. Betty Kamen and Si Kamen, "Kitchen Cupboard Skin Care," Filmstrip #26 (Burbank, CA.: Encore Visual Education, Inc., 1980).
40. Dian Dincin Buchman, *Herbal Medicine: The Natural Way to Get Well and Stay Well* (New York: David McKay Co., Inc., 1979), pp. 19–25.
41. G. Garamy, "Engineering Aspects of Cryosurgery," in *Cryosurgery*, eds. R. W. Rand et al. (Springfield, IL: Charles C. Thomas, Publishers, 1968).
42. Thomas Nashe, "In Time of Pestilence," in *Dictionary of Quotations*, ed. Bergen Evans, *op. cit.*, p. 49.
43. Fables, 1700, in *Dictionary of Quotations*, *op. cit.*
44. Problems and Solutions, "Postpartum Alopecia is Largely Untreatable But Almost Certainly Transient," *Postgraduate Medicine* 72 (September 1982):35.
45. Irwin I. Lubowe and Barbara Huss, *A Teenage Guide to Healthy Skin and Hair* (New York: E.P. Dutton, 1979), p. 85.
46. William Shakespeare, *Comedy of Errors*, act 2, scene 2.
47. Lubowe and Huss, *op. cit.*, pp. 77–78.
48. *Ibid.*
49. R. J. Cairins, "Metabolic and Nutritional Disorders," in *Textbook of Der-*

matology, 2nd ed., eds. A. Rook, D. S. Wilkinson, and F. J. G. Ebling (London: Blackwell Scientific Publications, 1972), pp. 1873–87.

50. Lubowe and Huss, *op. cit.*, p. 85.
51. Kunin, *op. cit.*, p. 56.
52. Lowell A. Goldsmith, "Vitamins and Alopecia," *Archives of Dermatology* 116 (July–December 1980):1135–36.
53. L. Sweetman, L. Suhr, and W. L. Nyhan, "Deficiencies of Propioyl-coa and 3-Methylcrotonyl-coa Carboxylases in a Patient with a Dietary Deficiency of Biotin," *Clinical Research* 27 (1979):118A.
54. J. F. Rosen et al., "Rickets with Alopecia: An Inborn Error of Vitamin D Metabolism," *Journal of Pediatrics* 94 (1979):729–35.
55. Alfred Gilman, "Androgens and Anabolic Steroids," in *The Pharmacologic Basis of Therapeutics* (New York: Macmillan, 1975):1459.
56. Anthony R. Zappacosta, "Reversal of Baldness in Patient Receiving Minoxidil for Hypertension," *New England Journal of Medicine* 303 (December 18, 1980):1480–81.
57. George Bernard Shaw, *Man and Superman*, act 4.
58. William Butler Yeats, *Adam's Curse*.
59. William Shakespeare, *King Lear*, act 3, scene 2.
60. Rose E. Frische, Grace Wyshak, and Larry Vincent, "Delayed Menarche and Amenorrhea in Ballet Dancers," *New England Journal of Medicine* 303 (July 3, 1980):17–19.
61. Editorial: Opinion and Comment: "Acne Diet Reconsidered," *Archives of Dermatology* 117 (April 1981):193–95.
62. Personal communication with Jonathan Zissmore, M.D., dermatologist, New York. Personal files of Betty and Si Kamen, Larkspur, CA.
63. Edward R. Brace, *A Popular Guide to Medical Language* (New York: Van Nostrand Reinhold Co., 1983), pp. 31–32.
64. Clinical records at The Stress Center, Huntington, N.Y., 1982–83.
65. Hans Braun, "Sonderdruck aus Heft," *Archive für Arzneitherapie* 1 (1981):47–77.
66. O. H. Braun, "Effect of Consumption of Human Milk and Other Formulas on Intestinal Bacterial Flora in Infants," in *Textbook of Gastroenterology and Nutrition in Infancy*, vol. 1, ed. Emanuel Lebenthal (New York: Raven Press, 1981), pp. 247–52.
67. David F. Horrobin and S. C. Cunnane, "Interactions Between Zinc, Essential Fatty Acids, and Prostaglandins: Relevance to Acrodermatitis Enteropathica, Total Parenteral Nutrition, the Glucagonoma Syndrome, Diabetes, Anorexia Nervosa and Sickle Cell Syndrome," *Medical Hypothesis* 6 (1980):277–96.
68. Anthony A. Albanese, *Current Topics in Nutrition and Disease: Nutrition for the Elderly*, vol. 3 (New York: Alan R. Liss, Inc., 1980), p. 142.
69. Kunin, *op cit.*, p. 54.
70. *Ibid.*, p. 55.

71. M. A. Crawford, "The Role of Essential Fatty Acids and Prostaglandins," *Postgraduate Medical Journal* 56 (August 1980):559–62.
72. C. Vergani et al., "Low Levels of HDL in Severe Cystic Acne," *New England Journal of Medicine* 307 (October 28, 1982):1151–52.
73. Editorial, "Retinoids in Dermatology," *Lancet* 1 (March 7, 1981):537–38.
74. Richard A. Pittsley and Frank W. Yoder, "Retinoid Hyperostosis: Skeletal Toxicity Associated with Long-term Administration of 13-Cis-Retinoic Acid for Refractory Ichthyosis," *New England Journal of Medicine* 308 (April 28, 1983):1012–14.
75. Peter E. Pochi, "Hormones, Retinoids, and Acne," *New England Journal of Medicine* 308 (April 28, 1983):1024–25.
76. A. Wagner and G. Plewig, "13 cis-Retinsause: Pharmakologische und toxikologische Untersuchungen bei der Behandlung Schwerster Akneformen," *Münchener Mediziniche Wochenschrift* 38 (1979):1294–1300.
77. S. Wright and J. L. Burton, "Oral Evening-Primrose-Seed Oil Improves Atopic Eczema," *Lancet* 1 (November 20, 1982):1120.
78. James Thomson, "Autumn," *The Seasons*, in *Dictionary of Quotations*, ed. Bergen Evans, *op. cit.*, p. 49.
79. Diogenes Laertius, "Aristotle," V 18, in *Dictionary of Quotations*, ed. Bergen Evans, *op. cit.*, p. 49.
80. Robert Neuhaus and Ruby Neuhaus, *Successful Aging* (New York: John Wiley and Sons, 1982), pp. 36–37.
81. Sharon Faelten, *The Complete Book of Minerals for Health* (Emmaus, PA: Rodale Press, 1981), pp. 86, 384–86.
82. Jeffrey Bland, Symposium, *op. cit.*
83. Wulf H. Utian, *Your Middle Years: A Doctor's Guide for Today's Woman* (Norwalk, CT: Appleton-Century-Crofts, 1980), p. 38.
84. Charles F. Wetherall, *Kicking the Coffee Habit* (Minneapolis: Wetherall Publishing Co., 1981), pp. 110–111.
85. Kunin, *op. cit.*, pp. 64–68.
86. Harold H. Sandstead, James P. Carter, and William J. Darby, "How to Diagnose Nutritional Deficiencies," *Nutrition Today* 4 (Summer 1969).
87. Interview with Joseph Consentino, M.D., plastic surgeon of Syosset, New York, WMCA Radio, New York, November 24, 1982.
88. Howard Bezoza, M.D., surgeon, personal communication, July 1983. Personal files of Betty and Si Kamen, Larkspur, CA.
89. T. K. Basu and C. J. Schorah, *Vitamin C in Health and Disease* (Westport, CT: AVI Publishing Co., 1982), p. 109.
90. Benjamin Franklin, *Poor Richard's Almanac* (1734).
91. Lubowe and Huss, *op. cit.*, pp. 80–81.
92. John Yudkin, *Sweet and Dangerous* (New York: Peter H. Wyden, Inc., 1972), p. 137.
93. "Alopecia of Nutritional and Metabolic Origin," in *Textbook of Der-

matology, 2nd ed., eds. A. Rook, D. S. Wilkinson, and F. J. G. Ebling (London: Blackwell Scientific Publications, 1972), pp. 1596–97.

94. *Compendium of Most Common Skin Disorders* (New York: Dome Chemicals, Inc., 1964), p. 24.
95. Stuart Maddin, *Current Dermatologic Management* (St. Louis: C. V. Mosby Company, 1970), p. 79.
96. *Ibid.,* p. 82.
97. Howard Bezoza, personal communication, *op. cit.*
98. Pfeiffer, *op. cit.,* p. 467.
99. Nonsense verse on hair.
100. Ruth Winter, *Cancer-Causing Agents* (New York: Herbert Michelman Book, Crown Publishers, 1979), pp. 67, 110–112.
101. Pfeiffer, *op. cit.,* p. 180.
102. *Ibid.*
103. Michael C. Archer and Steven R. Tannenbaum, "Vitamins," in *Nutritional and Safety Aspects of Food Processing,* ed. Steven R. Tannenbaum (New York: Marcel Dekker, Inc., 1979), p. 80.
104. G. H. Miller, "The Pennsylvania Study on Passive Smoking," *Journal of Breathing* 41 (1978):5–9.
105. T. Hirayama, "Non-Smoking Wives of Heavy Smokers Have a Higher Risk of Lung Cancer: A Study from Japan," *British Medical Journal* 282 (1981):183–85.
106. S. S. Stahl et al., "The Effects of Protein Deprivation Upon the Oral Tissues of the Rat and Particularly Upon the Periodontal Structures Under Irritation," *Oral Surgery, Oral Medicine, Oral Pathology* 8 (1955):760.
107. A. Sheehan, "The Prevalence and Severity of Periodontal Disease in Rural Nigerians," *Dental Practice* 17 (1966):51.
108. Abraham E. Nizel, *Nutrition in Preventive Dentistry* (Philadelphia: W. B. Saunders Co., 1981), p. 481.
109. *Ibid.,* p. 482.
110. Betty Kamen and Si Kamen, *Kids Are What They Eat* (New York: Arco Publishing Inc., 1983), pp. 143–44.
111. L. M. Screebny, "Effects of Physical Consistency of Food on the 'Crevicular Complex' and the Salivary Glands," *International Dental Journal* 22 (1972):394.
112. D. S. Larato, "Effects of Unilateral Mastication on Teeth and Periodontal Structures," *Journal of Oral Medicine* 25 (1970):80.
113. E. D. Coolidge, "The Thickness of the Human Periodontal Membrane," *Journal of the American Dental Association* 24 (1937):1260.
114. Kenneth Barlow, "Your Teeth All Your Life," *Nutrition and Health* 1 (1982):103–107.
115. A. Sheiham, "Sugar and Dental Decay," *Lancet* 1 (April 16, 1983):873.
116. Editorial, "Hot Peppers and Substance P," *Lancet* 1 (May 28, 1983):1198–99.

117. G. Isaacs, "Permanent Local Anesthesia and Anhidrosis After Clove Oil Spillage," *Lancet* 1 (April 16, 1983):882.
118. "The Nutrition Gazette," *Nutrition Today* (July-August 1982):3.

Chapter 3: The Scale Association

1. Judy Freespirit, Nancy Thomas, and Louise Wolf, Phil Donahue Program transcript #04063, 1983.
2. Joan Rivers, Johnny Carson Program, 1983.
3. J. S. Garrow et al., "Predisposition to Obesity," *Lancet* 1 (May 24, 1980):1103–4.
4. W. Wyrwicka, "The Problem of Motivation in Feeding Behavior," in *Hunger: Basic Mechanisms and Clinical Implications*, eds. D. Novin, W. Wyrwicka, and G. Bray (New York: Raven Press, 1976), pp. 203–13.
5. E. Mason, "Obesity in Pet Dogs," *Veterinary Record* 86 (1970):612–616.
6. Edward M. Stricker, "Hyperphagia," *New England Journal of Medicine* 298 (May 4, 1978):1010–13.
7. J. Magnen, "Advances in Studies on the Physiological Control and Regulation of Food Intake," in *Progress in Physiological Psychology*, vol. 4, eds. E. Stellar and J. M. Sprague (New York: Academic Press, 1971), pp. 203–261.
8. Jane E. Brody, "New Dieting Theory's Delicate Balance," *New York Times*, May 19, 1982, p. C1.
9. K. H. Sidney, R. J. Shepard, and J. Harrison, "Endurance Training and Body Composition of the Elderly," *American Journal of Clinical Nutrition* 30 (1977):326–33.
10. Emil Apfelbaum, "Pathophysiology of the Circulatory System in Hunger Disease," in *Hunger Disease*, ed. Myron Winick (New York: John Wiley and Sons, 1979), p. 134.
11. The patient-doctor interchange was based on interview with Serafina Corsello, M.D., Medical Director of The Stress Center in Huntington, N.Y., March 1983.
12. Editorial, "Do the Lucky Ones Burn Off Their Dietary Excesses?" *Lancet* 2 (November 24, 1979):1115–16.
13. J. R. K. Robson, "Metabolic Response to Food," *Lancet* 2 (December 24 & 31, 1977):1367.
14. Brody, *op. cit.*
15. J. Sonka, "Effects of Diet or Diet and Exercise in Weight Reducing Regimens," in *Nutrition, Physical Fitness, and Health*, eds. Jana Parizkova and V. A. Rogozkin (Baltimore: University Park Press, 1978), p. 239.
16. This account is summarized from Myron Winick, *Hunger Disease* (New York: John Wiley and Sons, 1979), pp. 39, 41, 72, 75, 127, 182, 200, 214–15, 219, 220, 222.
17. D. A. Booth, F. M. Toates, and S. V. Platt, "Control System for Hun-

ger and its Implications in Animals and Man," in *Hunger: Basic Mechanisms and Clinical Implications,* eds. D. Novin, W. Wyrwicka, and G. A. Bray (New York: Raven Press, 1976), pp. 127–143.

18. N. E. Rowland and S. M. Antelman, "Stress-Induced Hyperphagia and Obesity in Rats: A Possible Model for Understanding Human Obesity," *Science* 191 (1976):310–12.
19. Ancel Keys et al., *The Biology of Human Starvation* (Minneapolis: University of Minnesota Press, 1950), pp. 63–78, 843.
20. Horst Kather and Bernd Simon, "Opioid Peptides and Obesity," *Lancet* 2 (October 27, 1979):905.
21. Anne Ferguson, "Diagnosis and Treatment of Lactose Intolerance," *British Medical Journal* 283 (November 28, 1981):1423–24.
22. B. W. Martin, "Aspirin for Gluten Enteropathy," *Lancet* 2 (November 13, 1982):1099–1100.
23. R. Ferguson, G. K. T. Holmes, and W. T. Cooke, "Celiac Disease, Fertility, and Pregnancy," *Scandinavian Journal of Gastroenterology* 17 (1982):65–68.
24. Judith H. Dobrzynski, *Fasting: A Way to Well-Being* (New York: Sovereign Books, 1979), pp. 2–3.
25. William Dufty, *Sugar Blues* (Radnor, PA: Chilton Book Co., 1975), p. 100.
26. Stanley H. Title and Charles M. Klein, *Sensibly Thin* (Chicago: Nelson-Hall, 1979), pp. 78–81.
27. Jean Mayer, "Obesity," in *Modern Nutrition in Health and Disease,* eds. Robert S. Goodhart and Maurice E. Shils (Philadelphia: Lea and Febiger, 1980), p. 738.
28. E. J. Drenick, "Obesity in Perspective," *Fogarty International Center Series on Preventive Medicine,* 2 (1974):341.
29. Allan Cott, *Fasting: The Ultimate Diet* (New York: Bantam, 1975), p. 4.
30. Rafael Lantigua et al., "Cardiac Arrhythmias Associated With a Liquid Protein Diet for the Treatment of Obesity," *New England Journal of Medicine* 303 (1980):735–38.
31. Gerald J. Friedman, "Diet in Treatment of Diabetes Mellitus," in *Modern Nutrition in Health and Disease,* eds. Robert S. Goodhart and Maurice E. Shils (Philadelphia: Lea and Febiger, 1980), pp. 985–86.
32. D. Johnson and E. J. Drenick, "Therapeutic Fasting in Morbid Obesity," *Archives of Internal Medicine* 137 (1977):1381–82.
33. Richard Smith, *The Bronx Diet* (New York: Workman Publishing, 1979), p. 69.
34. P. A. Stefanik, F. P. Heald, and J. Mayer, "Caloric Intake in Relation to Energy Output of Obese and Nonobese Adolescent Boys," *American Journal of Clinical Nutrition* 7 (1959):55–62.
35. J. Mayer et al., "Relation Between Caloric Intake, Body Weight, and

Physical Work," *American Journal of Clinical Nutrition* 4 (1956):169–75.

36. J. Parizkova, "Body Composition and Lipid Metabolism in Relation to Nutrition and Exercise," in *Nutrition, Physical Fitness, and Health,* eds. Jana Parizkova and V. A. Rogozkin (Baltimore: University Park Press, 1978), p. 239.

37. J. Parizkova and L. Stankova, "Influence of Physical Activity on a Treadmill on the Metabolism of Adipose Tissue in Rats," *British Journal of Nutrition* 18 (1964):325–32.

38. J. Parizkova and E. Eiselt, "Body Composition and Anthropometric Indicators in Old Age and the Influence of Physical Exercise," *Human Biology* 38 (1966):351.

39. J. Suzuki et al., "Studies of the Nutrition of the Sportsman (Report2/0): Morphological Measurement of Sumo-Wrestlers," *Japanese Journal of Nutrition* 19 (1961):191.

40. J. Parizkova and R. Poledne, "Consequences of Long-Term Hypokinesia as Compared to Mild Exercise in Lipid Metabolism of the Heart, Skeletal Muscle, and Adipose Tissue," *European Journal of Applied Physiology* 33 (1974):331–38.

41. "Food and Obesity in the Rat," *Nutrition Reviews* 37 (February 1979):52–53.

42. Jeffrey Bland, Symposium: Nutritional Approaches to the Management of Intestinal Disorders, Autoimmune Phenomena, and Endocrinopathies, New York City, March 19 & 20, 1983.

43. Richard J. Wurtman, "Nutrition: The Changing Scene: Behavioral Effects of Nutrients," *Lancet* 1 (May 21, 1983):1145–47.

44. "Men, Women, and Obesity," *British Medical Journal* 4 (1974):249–50.

45. R. E. Nisbett, "Determinants of Food Intake in Obesity," *Science* 159 (1968):1254–55.

46. G. A. Leveille and D. R. Romsos, "Meal Eating and Obesity," *Nutrition Today* (November–December 1974).

47. W. P. T. James et al., "Elevated Metabolic Rates in Obesity," *Lancet* 1 (May 27, 1978):1122–25.

48. Fred A. Kummerow and Harlan E. Moore, "Saturated Fat and Cholesterol Dietary 'Risk Factors' or Essentials to Human Life?" *Food and Nutrition* 53 (September–October 1981):1–5.

49. A. Pradalier et al., "Pain and Obesity," *Lancet* 1 (May 17, 1980):1090–91.

50. Edward W. McDonagh, "Obesity: The American Tragedy," *Your Health* (April 1983):1–2.

51. *Ibid.*

52. Editorial, "Obesity: The Cancer Connection," *Lancet* 1 (May 29, 1982):1223–24.

53. Efrain Reisen et al., "Effect of Weight Loss Without Salt Restriction on

the Reduction of Blood Pressure in Overweight Hypertensive Patients," *New England Journal of Medicine* 298 (January 5, 1978):1–6.

54. R. J. Jarrett, "The Problems of Food Abundance," in *Nutrition and Disease*, ed. R. J. Jarrett (Baltimore: University Park Press, 1979), p. 140.
55. *Ibid.*
56. J. R. Thornton, "Gallstone Disappearance Associated with Weight Loss," *Lancet* 2 (September 1, 1979):478.
57. Patrick J. Bradley, "Diet and Coronary Heart Disease," *The Medical Journal of Australia* 1 (March 1980):285.
58. Jeffrey T. Wack and Judith Rodin, "Smoking and Its Effects on Body Weight and the Systems of Caloric Regulation," *The American Journal of Clinical Nutrition* 35 (February 1982):366–80.
59. Kenneth Phillips, "Zero in on Obesity," *Obesity-Bariatric Medicine* 9 (1980):126–27.
60. Marian Thompson Arlin, *The Science of Nutrition* (New York: Macmillan Publishing Co., 1972), p. 253.
61. Jean A. Pennington, *Dietary Nutrient Guide* (Westport, CT: The AVI Publishing Co., Inc., 1976), p. 209.
62. John M. Douglass and Sue Douglass, "Milk: That Human Kindness Stuff," *Your Health,* Newsletter of the International Academy of Preventive Medicine (May–June 1983):1.
63. Marshall Mandell and Fran Gare Mandell, *It's Not Your Fault You're Fat Diet* (New York: Harper and Row, 1983), pp. 13–14.
64. Mehl McDowell, "Appetite Control: An Addiction-Like Component in Overeating and Its Cure," *Obesity-Bariatric Medicine* 9 (1980):138–43.
65. Elena O. Nightingale and Frederick C. Robbins, "Saccharine and Society," *American Journal of Medicine* 71 (1981):9–12.
66. W. O'Hara et al., "Fat Loss in the Cold: A Controlled Study," *Journal of Applied Physiology* 46 (1979):872–77.
67. Arlin, *op. cit.*
68. Sir John Suckling, "Of Thee, Kind Boy," *Fragmenta Aurea*, stanza 3 (1646), *Bartlett's Familiar Quotations*, centennial edition, ed. John Bartlett (Boston: Little, Brown and Co., 1955), p. 261b.
69. Edna St. Vincent Millay, *Figs From Thistles, First Fig, Bartlett's Familiar Quotations*, centennial edition, ed. John Bartlett (Boston: Little, Brown and Co., 1955), p. 962a.

Chapter 4: Food Consequences

1. Walter Yellowlees, "Nutrition, Health and the Future," *Nutrition and Health* 1 (1982):118–23.
2. William Shakespeare, *Romeo and Juliet* act 3, scene 2, line 83.
3. Oliver Goldsmith, *The Deserted Village.*

4. C. V. Jacks and R. White, *The Rape of the Earth* (London: Faber and Faber, 1951).

5. N. S. Scrimshaw, "Nature of Protein Requirements," *Journal of the American Dietetic Association* 54 (1969):94.

6. A. T. Mendeloff, "Dietary Fiber and Human Health," *New England Journal of Medicine* 297 (1977):811.

7. T. G. Kiehm, J. W. Anderson, and K. Ward, "Beneficial Effects of a High Carbohydrate, High Fiber Diet on Hyperglycemic Diabetic Men," *American Journal of Clinical Nutrition* 29 (1976):895.

8. B. K. Armstrong et al., "Hematological, Vitamin B_{12}, and Folate Studies in Seventh Day Adventist Vegetarians," *American Journal of Clinical Nutrition* 27 (1974):712.

9. E. C. Barton-Wright and W. A. Elliott, "The Pantothenic Acid Metabolism of Rheumatoid Arthritis," *Lancet* 2 (1963):862.

10. C. R. Sirtori et al., "Soybean-Protein Diet in the Treatment of Type-II Hyperlipoproteinemia," *Lancet* 1 (1977):275–77.

11. F. R. Ellis and T. A. B. Sanders, "Angina and Vegan Diet," *American Heart Journal* 1 (1977):803–5.

12. Rudolph Ballentine, *Diet and Nutrition: A Holistic Approach* (Honesdale, PA: The Himalayan International Institute, 1978), p. 98.

13. Beatrice Trum Hunter, *The Great Nutrition Robbery* (New York: Charles Scribner's Sons, 1978), pp. 67–70.

14. Jeffrey Bland, *Your Health Under Siege: Using Nutrition to Fight Back* (Brattleboro, VT: The Stephen Greene Press, 1981), pp. 75–76.

15. A. N. Howard and J. Marks, "The Lack of Evidence for a Hypocholesterolemic Factor in Milk," *Atherosclerosis* 45 (1982):243–47.

16. G. V. Mann, "Current Concepts: Diet-Heart End of an Era," *New England Journal of Medicine* 297 (1977):644–50.

17. David J. Roberts, "Butter," *Lancet* 1 (April 23, 1983):929–30.

18. E. B. Smith, "Atherogenicity and the Supermarket Shelf," *Lancet* 1 (1980):534.

19. J. A. L. Gorringe, "Butter," *Lancet* 1 (May 21, 1983):1165.

20. Kurt A. Oster, "Atherosclerosis: Conjectures, Data and Facts," *Nutrition Today* (November–December 1981):28–29.

21. Hunter, *op. cit.*, pp. 44–47.

22. Brent A. Blue, "The Stress of Playing God," *New England Journal of Medicine* 309 (July 21, 1983):193.

23. D. Deykin, P. Janson, and L. McMahon, "Ethanol Potentiation of Aspirin-Induced Prolongation of the Bleeding Time," *New England Journal of Medicine* 306 (1982):852–54.

24. B. Brantmark, "Salicylate Inhibition of Antiplatelet Effect of Aspirin," *Lancet* 2 (December 12, 1981):1349.

25. H. W. Davenport, "Gastric Mucosal Hemorrhage in Dogs: Effects of Acid,

Aspirin and Alcohol," *Gastroenterology* 56 (1969):439–49.

26. C. H. Morris et al., "Effect of Aspirin and Ethanol on the Gastric Mucosa of the Rat," *Journal of Pharmacological Science* 61 (1972):815–18.

27. Marshal Shlafer, "Aspirin and Alcohol," *New England Journal of Medicine* 307 (October 7, 1982):951.

28. Robert J. Peshek, "Clinical Nutrition for Universities?" *Journal of Applied Nutrition* 30 (1978):1.

29. Rashi Fein, *Sounding Boards,* "What is Wrong with the Language of Medicine?" *New England Journal of Medicine* 306 (April 8, 1982):863–64.

30. Derrick Lonsdale, "Thou Shalt Do No Harm" *International Journal of Biosocial Research* 4 (1983):107–14.

31. N. K. Clapp, L. C. Satterfield, and N. D. Bowles, "Effects of the Antioxidant Butylated Hydroxytoluene (BHT) on Mortality in Balb/c Mice," *Journal of Gerontology* 34 (1979):497–501.

32. Denham Harman and Noffsinger, "Free Radical Theory of Aging: Inhibition of Amyloidosis in Mice by Antioxidants; Possible Mechanism," *Journal of the American Geriatric Society* 23 (1976):203–209.

33. Edward J. Calabrese, *Nutrition and Environmental Health: The Influence of Nutritional Status on Pollutant Toxicity and Carcinogenicity* (New York: Wiley-Interscience Publication, 1981), pp. 456–57.

34. J. Stokes, C. L. Scudder, and A. G. Karczmar, "Effects of Chronic Treatment with Established Food Preservatives on Brain Chemistry and Behavior of Mice," *Federation Proceedings* 31 (1972):596.

35. J. Stokes and C. L. Scudder, "The Effects of Butylated Hydroxytoluene on Behavioral Development of Mice," *Developmental Psychobiology* 7 (1974):343–50.

36. Durk Pearson and Sandy Shaw, *Life Extension: A Practical Scientific Approach* (New York: Warner Books, 1982), p. 369.

37. Stephen Levine, Ph.D., Director of the Allergy Research Group, Concord, CA. Personal communication, August 1983. Personal files of Betty and Si Kamen, Larkspur, CA.

38. Carl C. Pfeiffer, *Mental and Elemental Nutrients: A Physician's Guide to Nutrition and Health Care* (New Canaan, CT: Keats Publishing, Inc., 1975), p. 47.

39. Beatrice Trum Hunter, *Food Additives and Federal Policy: The Mirage of Safety* (New York: Charles Scribner's Sons, 1975), pp. 134–35.

40. Lenhart Juhlin, "Incidence of Intolerance to Food Additives," *International Journal of Dermatology* 19 (December 1980):548–51.

41. Hunter, *Food Additives,* op. cit., p. 136.

42. O. Meyers and E. Hansen, "Behavioral and Developmental Effects of Butylated Hydroxytoluene Dosed Rats in Utero and in the Lactation Period," *Toxicology* 16 (1980):247–58.

43. C. V. Vorhees et al., "Developmental Neurobehavioral Toxicity of Butylated Hydroxytoluene in Rats," *Food Cosmetics and Toxicology* 19 (1981):153–62.
44. Pearson and Shaw, *op. cit.*, pp. 751–52.
45. H. Babich, "Butylated Hydroxytoluene (BHT): A Review," *Environmental Research* 29 (1982):1–29.
46. Hunter, *Food Additives, op. cit.*, p. 136.
47. *Ibid.*, p. 119.
48. Pearson and Shaw, *op. cit.*, p. 391.
49. Hunter, *Food Additives, op. cit.*, p. 112.
50. Pearson and Shaw, *op. cit.*, p. 102.
51. G. B. Haber, K. W. Heaton, and D. Murphy, "Depletion and Disruption of Dietary Fiber," *Lancet 2* (October 1, 1977):679–82.
52. R. Q. Frazier et al., "Atherogenesis in the Cebus Monkey. 1. A Comparison of Three Food Fats Under Controlled Dietary Conditions," *Archives of Pathology* 74 (1962):312–22.
53. D. Vesselinovitch, "Atherosclerosis in the Rhesus Monkey Fed Three Food Fats," *Atherosclerosis* 20 (1974):303–21.
54. D. S. Grimes and C. Gordon, "Satiety Value of Wholemeal and White Bread," *Lancet 2* (July 8, 1978):106.
55. Editorial, "Dietary Dogma Disproved," *Science* 220 (April 29, 1983):487–88.
56. L. Patrick Coyle, *The World Encyclopedia of Food* (New York: Facts on File, Inc., 1982), p. 161.
57. "Eat a Chick Pea Today," *Soil and Health News* 11 (February 1982):2.
58. "Amino Acid Content of Foods," *Home Economics Research* Report #4, United States Department of Agriculture, 1968.
59. "Interaction Between Methionine, Fat and Choline in the Young Rat," *Journal of Nutrition* 100 (June 1970):664–70.
60. "Nutritional Significance of Dietary Imbalance," *Federation Proceedings* 23 (1963):1059.
61. Betty Kamen and Si Kamen, *Kids Are What They Eat: What Every Parent Needs to Know About Nutrition* (New York: Arco Publishing, Inc., 1983), p. 161.
62. "Nutrition and Cancer: A Matter of Prudence," *Courier* 4 (January 1981):2–3.
63. L. W. Wattenberg et al., "Dietary Constituents Altering the Responses to Chemical Carcinogens," *Federation Proceedings* 35 (1976):1327.
64. J. Lawrence Werther, "Food and Cancer," *New York State Journal of Medicine* 80 (August 1980):1401–7.
65. Sanford J. Kempin, "Warfarin Resistance Caused by Broccoli," *New England Journal of Medicine* 308 (May 19, 1983):1229.
66. Betty Kamen and Si Kamen, "Vegetarianism: Healthful Eating," Film-

strip #20 (Burbank, CA: Encore Visual Education, Inc., 1980).

67. M. B. Sporn and D. L. Newton, *Federation Proceedings* 38 (1979):2528–34.

68. N. Wald et al., "Low-Serum-Vitamin-A and Subsequent Risk of Cancer, *Lancet* 2 (October 18, 1980):813–15.

69. J. D. Kark et al., "Serum Vitamin A (Retinal) and Cancer Incidence in Evans County, Georgia," *Journal of the National Cancer Institute* 66 (1981):7–16.

70. C. Mettlin, S. Graham, and M. Swanson, "Vitamin A and Lung Cancer," *Journal of the National Cancer Institute* 62 (1979):1435–38.

71. M. P. Vessey, K. McPherson, and D. Yeates, "Mortality in Oral Contraceptive Users," letter to *Lancet* 1 (March 7, 1981):549–50.

72. P. M. Layde and V. Beral, "Further Analyses of Mortality in Oral Contraceptive Users, letter to *Lancet* 1 (March 7, 1981):541–46.

73. Coyle, *op. cit.*, p. 136.

74. Emil Ginter, "Optimum Intake of Vitamin C for the Human Organism," *Nutrition and Health* 1 (1982):66–77.

75. R. E. Hughes, R. J. Hurley, and E. Jones, "Dietary Ascorbic Acid and Muscle Carnitine (b-OH-y-Trimethylamino Butyric Acid) in Guinea Pigs," *British Journal of Nutrition* 43 (1980):385–87.

76. E. Ginter, P. Bobek, and D. Vargova, "Tissue Levels and Optimum Dosage of Vitamin C in Guinea Pigs," *Nutrition and Metabolism* 23 (1979):217–26.

77. O. Cerna and E. Ginter, "Blood Lipids and Vitamin C Status," *Lancet* 1 (May 13, 1978):1055–56.

78. Emil Ginter *op. cit.*, "Optimum Intake of Vitamin C for the Human Organism," *Nutrition and Health* 1 (1982):66–77.

79. T. K. Basu and C. J. Schorah, *Vitamin C in Health and Disease* (Westport, CT: AVI Publishing Co., 1982), p. 53.

80. B. Leibovitz and B. V. Siegel, "Ascorbic Acid and the Immune Response," in *Diet and Resistance to Disease: Advances in Experimental Medicine and Biology*, eds. Marshall Phillips and Albert Baetz (New York: Plenum Press, 1981), p. 9.

81. *Ibid.*, p. 18.

82. B. L. Murphy et al., "Ascorbic Acid and Its Effects on Parainfluenza Type III Virus Infection in Cotton-Topped Marmosets," *Laboratory Animal Science* 24 (1974):229–32.

83. A. Murata et al., "Mechanism of Inactivation of Bacteriophage Delt-A Containing Single-Stranded DNA by Ascorbic Acid," *Journal of Nutrition Science: Vitaminology* 21 (1975):261–69.

84. S. Banic, "Prevention of Rabies by Vitamin C," *Nature* 258 (1975):153–54.

85. Joanne Moyer, *Nuts and Seeds: The Natural Snacks* (Emmaus, PA: Rodale Press, 1973), pp. 56–57.

86. Steven R. Tannenbaum, "Vitamins and Minerals," in *Principles of Food Science: Food Chemistry*, Part 1, ed. Owen R. Fennema (New York: Marcel Dekker, Inc., 1976), p. 370.

87. Interview with Madhur Jaffrey, WMCA Radio, New York, June 16, 1982.

88. Barbara Griggs, *Green Pharmacy: A History of Herbal Medicine* (New York: The Viking Press, 1981), p. 13.

89. Betty Kamen and Si Kamen, "Beans, Beans, Beans," Filmstrip #201 (Burbank, CA: Encore Visual Education, Inc., 1981).

90. Thomas R. Dawber, "Eggs, Serum Cholesterol, and Coronary Heart Disease," *American Journal of Clinical Nutrition* 36 (October 1982):617–25.

91. American Medical Association Release, October 12, 1962.

92. Mann, *op. cit.*, p. 644.

93. Edward R. Gruberg and Stephen A. Raymond, *Beyond Cholesterol* (New York: St. Martin's Press, 1981), p. 30.

94. Allen B. Nicols et al., "Independence on Serum Lipid Levels," *Journal of the American Medical Association* 236 (October 1976):1948–53.

95. A. Kamio, F. A. Kummerow, and H. Imai, "Degeneration of Aortic Smooth Muscle Cells in Swine Fed Excess Vitamin D₃," *Archives of Pathological Laboratory Medicine* 101 (1977):378.

96. Pfeiffer, *op. cit.*, pp. 81–87.

97. Betty Kamen and Si Kamen, "Grain Cookery," Filmstrip #21 (Burbank, CA: Encore Visual Education, Inc., 1980).

98. Coyle, *op. cit.*, p. 145.

99. *Ibid.*, p. 560.

100. June Armstrong, *Pick Your Poison: A Dictionary of Food Additives* (North Hollywood: Model Printing, 1973), p. 99.

101. William Kropf and Milton Houben, *Harmful Food Additives: The Eat Safe Guide* (Port Washington, NY: Ashley Books, Inc., 1980), p. 63.

102. Hunter, *Food Additives*, *op. cit.*, p. 92.

103. Television Presentation, "Sixty Minutes," NBC, February 13, 1983.

104. Joan Gussow, Professor, Columbia University, lecture at Jo Giese Brown Symposium, New York, June 23, 1981.

105. Lenhart Juhlin, "Incidence of Intolerance to Food Additives," *International Journal of Dermatology* 19 (December 1980):548–51.

106. Richard G. Cutler, "The Dysdifferentiative Hypothesis of Mammalian Aging and Longevity," in *Aging: The Aging Brain: Cellular and Molecular Mechanisms of Aging in the Nervous System* (New York: Raven Press, 1982), pp. 1–19.

107. W. A. Gortner, "The Impact of Food Technology on Nutrient Supplies," *Food Technology of Australia* 24 (1972):504–17.

108. Dietrich Knorr, "The Influence of Food Processing on the Nutritional Quality of Food," in *Soil, Food and Health in a Changing World*, eds.

Kenneth Barlow and Peter Bunyard (London: AB Academic Publishers, 1981), pp. 38–39.

109. Beatrice Trum Hunter, *Consumer Beware* (New York: Simon and Schuster, 1971), pp. 244–45.

110. M. Morita and M. Fujimaki, *Agriculture Food Chemistry* 21 (1973):860.

111. L. H. Going, *Journal of the American Oil Chemists' Society* 45 (1968):632.

112. A. Vioque et al., *Journal of the American Oil Chemists' Society* 42 (1965):344.

113. Lloyd A. Witting, Edward G. Perkins, and Fred A. Kummerow, "Lipids," in *Nutritional and Safety Aspects of Food Processing,* ed. Steven R. Tannenbaum (New York: Marcel Dekker, Inc., 1979), p. 114.

114. Ruth Winter, *Cancer-Causing Agents: A Preventive Guide* (New York: Crown Publishers, 1979), p. 160.

115. A. D. Rich and A. Greentree, *Journal of the American Oil Chemists' Society* 35 (1958):284.

116. G. Van Den Bosch, *Journal of the American Oil Chemists' Society* 50 (1973):487.

117. G. R. List et al., *Journal of the American Oil Chemists' Society* 44 (1967):485.

118. Bonnie F. Liebman and Sidney Wolfe, "Nutritive Value of Processed Meats," *New England Journal of Medicine* 307 (July 15, 1982):191.

119. Committee on Dietary Allowances, Food and Nutrition Board. Recommended Dietary Allowances. Washington, D.C. National Academy of Sciences, 1980.

120. Jim Mason and Peter Singer, *Animal Factories* (New York: Crown Publishers, Inc., 1980), p. 12.

121. *Ibid.,* p. 54.

122. M. A. Crawford, "A Re-Evaluation of the Nutrient Role of Animal Products," in *Proceedings of the III World Conference on Animal Production,* ed. R.L. Reid (Sydney: Sydney University Press, 1975), p. 24.

123. Deborah Danoff et al., "Big Mac Attack," *New England Journal of Medicine* 298 (May 11, 1978):1095.

124. International Agency for Research on Cancer. Sex Hormones II. I.A.R.C. Monographs on the Evaluation of the Carcinogenic Risk of Chemicals to Humans, vol. 21 (Lyon: I.A.R.C., 1979).

125. Editorial, "Anabolics in Meat Production," *Lancet* 1 (March 27, 1982):721–22.

126. Barbara M. Shannon and Sara C. Parks, "Fast Foods: A Perspective on Their Nutritional Impact," *Journal of the American Dietetic Association* 76 (March 1980):242–47.

127. E.H. Martin, "Food Protection in the 1980s," *Restaurant Business* 76 (December 1977):94.

128. Ross Hume Hall, "A Cell's Eye View of the Four Food Groups and Agricultural Policy," *Nutrition and Health* 1 (1982):20–23.

129. Bonnie Liebman, "Picking the Best and the Worst of Fast Food Offerings," *Nutrition Action* 10 (July–August 1983):19.
130. Jeffrey Bland, "Metabolic Update," Bellevue–Redmont Clinic, WA, July 1983. Tape series.
131. "Possible Vitamin B$_6$ Deficiency Uncovered in Persons with the 'Chinese Restaurant Syndrome,' " *Nutrition Reviews* 40 (January 1982):15–16.
132. David Sheinkin, Michael Schachter, and Richard Hutton, *The Food Connection: How the Things You Eat Affect the Way You Feel and What You Can Do About It* (New York: Bobbs-Merrill Co., Inc., 1979), p. 32.
133. David H. Allen and Gary J. Baker, "Chinese-Restaurant Asthma," *New England Journal of Medicine* 305 (November 5, 1981):1154–55.
134. K. Folkers et al., "Biochemical Evidence for a Deficiency of Vitamin B$_6$ in Subjects Reacting to the Monosodium-L-glutamate by the Chinese Restaurant Syndrome," *Biochemical Biophysics Research Communication* 100 (1981):972–77.
135. Pfeiffer, *op. cit.*, p. 40.
136. Hunter, *Food Additives, op. cit.*, p. 95.
137. *Ibid.*, p. 208.
138. Interview with Beatrice Trum Hunter, WMCA Radio, New York, November 30, 1980.
139. Donald R. Davis, "Nutrition in the United States: Much Room for Improvement," *Journal of Applied Nutrition* 35 (1983):17–29.
140. Warren Levin, M.D., Director of the World Health Medical Group, New York, personal communication, July 1983. "What's the Story on Fats?" Personal files of Betty and Si Kamen, Larkspur CA.
141. Anonymous Poem.
142. Michael deCourcy Hinds, "Assessing Effects of Chemically Treated Food," *New York Times*, March 31, 1982, p. C-1.
143. H. M. Sinclair, "The Diet of Canadian Indians and Eskimos," *Proceedings of the Nutrition Society* 12 (1953):69–82.
144. H. M. Sinclair, "Nutrition and Atherosclerosis," *Symposium of the Zoological Society of London* 21 (1968):275–88.
145. Editorial, "Eskimo Diets and Diseases," *Lancet* 1 (May 21, 1983):1139–41.
146. J. L. Beare-Rogers, "Docosenoic Acids in Dietary Fats," *Progress in Chemical Fats and Other Lipids* 15 (1977):29–56.
147. Coyle, *op. cit.*, p. 367.
148. James B. Young and Lewis Landsberg, "Effect of Oral Sucrose on Blood Pressure in the Spontaneously Hypertensive Rat," *Metabolism* 30 (May 1981):421–24.
149. Nancy A. Marlin and Theresa E. Cunningham, "Influence of Dietary Sugar on the Activity Levels of Preweanling Rats," *Journal of Applied Nutrition* 35 (1983):6–13.

150. Beatrice Trum Hunter, *The Sugar Trap and How to Avoid It* (Boston: Houghton Mifflin Co., 1982), p. 17.
151. Carl C. Pfeiffer and Jane Banks, *Dr. Pfeiffer's Total Nutrition* (New York: Simon and Schuster, 1980), p. 37.
152. *Ibid.*, p. 43.
153. R. J. Jarrett, "The Problems of Food Abundance," *Nutrition and Disease,* ed. R. J. Jarrett (Baltimore: University Park Press, 1979), p. 143.
154. W. J. Oliver, "Sodium Homeostasis and Low Blood Pressure Populations," in *Epidemiology of Arterial Blood Pressure,* eds. H. Kesteloot and J. U. Joossens (The Hague, The Netherlands: Martinus Nijhoff Publishers, 1980), pp. 229–41.
155. L. Ambard and E. Beaujard, "Causes de l' Hypertension Arterielle," *Archive of General Medicine* 1 (1904):520.
156. Report of the Senate Select Committee on Nutrition and Human Needs, "Dietary Goals of the United States" (Washington, D.C.: Government Printing Office, 1977):48–51.
157. J. M. Weiffenbach, P. A. Daniel, and B. J. Cowart, "Saltines in Developmental Perspective," in *Biological and Behavioral Aspects of Salt Intake,* eds. M. R. Kare, M. J. Fregly, and R. A. Bernard (New York: Academic Press, 1980), pp. 13–29.
158. W. J. Oliver, E. L. Cohen, and J. V. Neel, "Blood Pressure, Sodium Intake and Sodium Related Hormones in the Yanomama Indians: A 'No Salt' Culture," *Circulation* 52 (1975):146–51.
159. "FDA Issues Rules on Sodium Labeling," *Community Nutrition Institute* 12 (February 4, 1982):6.
160. Geoffrey H. Kalish, "Headaches After Red Wine," letter to *Lancet* 1 (June 6, 1981):1263.
161. E. R. Trethewie, "Wines and Headaches," *Medical Journal of Australia* 1 (1979):94.
162. Herbert Kaufman, "Headaches After Red Wine," letter to *Lancet* 1 (June 6, 1981):1263.

Chapter 5: The Stress Effect

1. Serafina Corsello, "Stress and Micronutrient Malabsorption," presented at the First Forum of Nutritional Medicine, San Francisco, March 1983. Researched by Serafina Corsello and Betty Kamen.
2. Tom Cox, *Stress* (Baltimore: University Park Press, 1978), pp. 50–51.
3. Marco Ermini, "Aging As A Biological Process: A Perspective," in *Aging, Immunity, and Arthritic Disease,* vol. 11, eds. Marguerite M. B. Kay, Jeffrey Galpin, and Takashi Makinodan (New York: Raven Press, 1980), p. 8.

4. *Dorland's Illustrated Medical Dictionary*, 25th edition (Philadelphia: W. B. Saunders, 1974), p. 754.
5. Richard J. Wurtman, "Nutrients That Modify Brain Function," *Scientific American* 246 (April 1982):50–59.
6. David J. Greenblatt and Richard I. Shader, "Drug Therapy: Current Status of Benzodiazepines," part 1, *New England Journal of Medicine* 309 (August 11, 1983):354–58.
7. J. O. Cole, D. S. Haskell, and M. H. Orzack, "Problems with the Benzodiazepines: An Assessment of the Available Evidence," *McLean Hospital Journal* 6 (1981):46–74.
8. K. Rickels, "Are Benzodiazepines Overused and Abused?" *British Journal of Clinical Pharmacology* 11, supplement (1981):71s–83s.
9. L. Lasagna, "The Halcion Story: Trial by Media," *Lancet* 1 (1980):815–16.
10. E. Bargmann et al., "Stopping Valium," *Public Citizen's Health Research Group*, Washington, D.C., 1982.
11. Joseph G. Chusid, *Correlative Neuroanatomy and Functional Neurology* (Los Altos, CA: Lange Medical Publications, 1970), p. 154.
12. Hans Selye, *The Stress of Life* (New York: McGraw-Hill Book Co., 1976), pp. 273–76.
13. Emerson Puch, quoted in *Lancet* 1 (February 19, 1983):398.
14. Bruce Smoller and Brian Schulman, *Pain Control: The Bethesda Program* (Garden City, NY: Doubleday and Co., Inc., 1982), pp. 39–41.
15. Olli Vuolteenaho, Juhani Leppaluoto, and Peka Mannisto, "Effect of Stress and Dexamethasone on Immunoreactive B-endorphin Levels in Rat Hypothalamus and Pineal," *Acta Physiologica Scandinavica* 114 (1982):7.
16. Hans Selye, personal communication, May, 1979. Personal files of Betty and Si Kamen, Larkspur CA.
17. Jeffrey Bland, *Your Health Under Siege: Using Nutrition to Fight Back* (Brattleboro, VT: The Stephen Greene Press, 1981), p. 97.
18. *Ibid.*
19. Don Mannerberg and June Roth, *Aerobic Nutrition* (New York: Hawthorn-Dutton, 1981), p. 25.
20. John M. Cleghorn, George Peterfy, and Emery J. Pinter, "Psychophysiology of Lipid Mobilization," in *Progress in Human Nutrition*, vol. 1, ed. Sheldon Margen (Westport, CT: AVI Publishing Co., 1971), p. 170.
21. Roslyn B. Alfin-Slater and Lilla Aftergood, "Lipids," in *Modern Nutrition In Health and Disease*, eds. Robert S. Goodhart and Maurice E. Shils (Philadelphia: Lea and Febiger, 1980), p. 124.
22. Mildred S. Seelig, *Magnesium Deficiency in the Pathogenesis of Disease: Early Roots of Cardiovascular, Skeletal, and Renal Abnormalities* (New York: Plenum Medical Book Co., 1980), p. 196.
23. Jeffrey Bland, *op. cit.*, p. 140.

24. John B. Jemmott III et al., "Academic Stress, Power Motivation, and Decrease in Secretion Rate of Salivary Secretory Immunoglobulin A," *Lancet* 1 (June 25, 1983):1400–2.
25. B.S. Dohrenwend and B.P. Dohrenwend, *Stressful Life Events: Their Nature and Effects* (New York: John Wiley, 1974).
26. M. Borysenko et al., "Stress and Dental Caries in the Rat," *Journal of Behavioral Medicine* 3 (1980):233–43.
27. S. V. Kasl, A. S. Evans, and J. C. Neiderman, "Psychosocial Risk Factors in the Development of Infectious Mononucleosis," *Psychosomatic Medicine* 41 (1979):445–66.
28. Hans Selye, *op. cit.*, p. 431.
29. Hans Selye, "Self-Regulation: The Response to Stress," in *Inner Balance: The Power of Holistic Healing*, ed. Elliott M. Goldwag (Englewood Cliffs, NJ: Prentice-Hall, Inc., 1979), pp. 66–68.
30. John H. Growdon, "Neurotransmitter Precursors in the Diet: Their Use in the Treatment of Brain Disease," in *Nutrition and the Brain*, vol. 3, eds. Richard J. Wurtman and Judith J. Wurtman (New York: Raven Press, 1979), p. 143.
31. John D. Kirschmann, *Nutrition Almanac* (New York: McGraw-Hill Book Co., 1975), p. 182.
32. Carl E. Anderson, "Vitamins," in *Nutritional Support of Medical Practice*, eds. Howard A. Schneider, Carl E. Anderson, and David B. Coursin (Hagerstown, MD: Medical Department, Harper and Row, Publishers, 1977), p. 53.
33. Carl C. Pfeiffer, *Mental and Elemental Nutrients: A Physician's Guide to Nutrition and Health Care* (New Canaan, CT: Keats Publishing, Inc., 1975), p. 130.
34. *Ibid.*, p. 129.
35. *Ibid.*, p. 133.
36. Interview with Irwin Stone, WMCA Radio, New York, November 21, 1981.
37. Kirschmann, *op. cit.*, p. 82.
38. Anderson, "Vitamins," *op. cit.*, p. 38.
39. Growdon, *op. cit.*, p. 143.
40. Smoller and Schulman, *op. cit.*, p. 29.
41. Growdon, *op. cit.*, p. 140.
42. Theodore L. Sourkes, "Nutrients and the Cofactors Required for Monoamine Synthesis in Nervous Tissue," in *Nutrition and the Brain*, vol. 3, eds. Richard J. Wurtman and Judith J. Wurtman (New York: Raven Press, 1979), p. 266.
43. Kirschmann, *op. cit.*, pp. 223–29.
44. Ford Heritage, *Composition and Facts About Food* (Mokelumne Hill, CA: Health Research, 1968), p. 92.

45. Pfeiffer, *op. cit.*, p. 226.
46. *Ibid.*, p. 230.
47. Kirschmann, *op. cit.*
48. Anderson, "Minerals," *op. cit.*, p. 67.
49. Kirschmann, *op. cit.*, p. 182.
50. Anderson, "Vitamins," *op. cit.*, p. 36.
51. Mark D. Altschule, *Nutritional Factors in General Medicine* (Springfield, IL: Charles C. Thomas, 1978), pp. 78–79.
52. Kirschmann, *op. cit.*
53. Altschule, *op. cit.*, p. 56.
54. Anderson, "Minerals," *op. cit.*, p. 64.
55. William H. Philpott and Dwight K. Kalita, *Brain Allergies: The Psychonutrient Connection* (New Canaan, CT: Keats Publishing, Inc., 1980), p. 61.
56. Seelig, *op. cit.*, p. 153.
57. *Ibid.*, p. 176.
58. Carlton Fredericks, *Carlton Fredericks' Program for Living Longer* (New York: Simon & Schuster, 1983), p. 100.
59. Anderson, "Minerals," *op. cit.*, p. 63.
60. Seelig, *op. cit.*, p. 224.
61. *Dorland's Illustrated Medical Dictionary*, *op. cit.*, p. 970.
62. Lot B. Page, "Nutritional Determinants of Hypertension," *Nutrition and the Killer Diseases* (New York: John Wiley & Sons, 1981), pp. 113–126.
63. Betty Kamen and Si Kamen, *The Kamen Plan for Total Nutrition During Pregnancy* (Norwalk, CT: Appleton-Century-Crofts, 1981), pp. 138–39.
64. Kirschmann, *op. cit.*, p. 183.
65. Carlton Fredericks, *Nutrition Guide for the Prevention and Cure of Common Ailments and Diseases* (New York: Simon & Schuster, 1982), p. 77.
66. Mannerberg and Roth, *op. cit.*, p. 37.
67. Charles F. Stroebel, *QR: The Quieting Reflex* (New York: G.P. Putnam's Sons, 1982), pp. 180–81.
68. Hans Selye, *Inner Balance*, p. 59.

Chapter 6: Specifics for the Pursuit of Youth

1. Clinical experience at The Stress Center, Huntington, New York.
2. Optimal diet prepared for The Stress Center, Huntington, New York, by Betty Karmen.
3. Seven-Day Meal and Menu Plan prepared for gluten- and wheat-sensitive patients at The Stress Center, Huntington, New York, by Betty Karmen.
4. Betty Kamen and Si Kamen, *The Kamen Plan for Total Nutrition During Pregnancy* (Norwalk, CT: Appleton-Century-Crofts, 1981), pp. 178–80.

5. Denis Burkitt, *Eat Right to Stay Healthy and Enjoy Life More* (New York: Arco Publishing, Inc., 1979), pp. 46–50.
6. David Horrobin, "Loss of Delta-6-Desaturase Activity As a Key Factor in Aging," *Medical Hypotheses* 7 (1981):1211–20.
7. M. G. Brush, "Efamol in the Treatment of the Premenstrual Syndrome," paper #9, Department of Gynecology, St. Thomas's Hospital Medical School, London.
8. Interview with David Horrobin, M.D., WMCA Radio, New York. June a40a981.
9. David Horrobin, *Medical Hypotheses, op. cit.*, p. 1217.
10. Interview with Diana Dalton, M.A., WMCA Radio, New York, September 21, 1980.

Chapter 7: Immunity and the Pursuit of Youth

1. T. Watts, "Thymus Weights in Malnourished Children," Journal of Tropical Pediatrics 15 (1969):155.
2. Tom Cox, *Stress* (Baltimore: University Park Press, 1978), p. 6.
3. Hans Selye, "Thymus and Adrenals in the Response of the Organisms to Injuries and Intoxications," *British Journal of Experimental Pathology* 17 (1936):234–48.
4. H. McFarlane and M. R. C. Path, "Malnutrition and Immunity," in *Immunological Aspects of Foods*, ed. Nicholas Catsimpoolas (Westport, CT: AVI Publishing Co., 1977), p. 373.
5. Edward R. Brace, *A Popular Guide to Medical Language* (New York: Van Nostrand Reinhold Co., 1983), p. 153.
6. C. T. Smith, American Council for the Association of Clinical Nutrition, Certification Course, module 1, tape 1, Clayton University, St. Louis, 1982.
7. Elisha Atkins, "Fever: New Perspective on an Old Phenomenon," *New England Journal of Medicine* 308 (April 21, 1983):958–59.
8. G. W. Duff and S. K. Durum, "Fever and Immunoregulation: Hyperthermia, Interleukins 1 and 2, and T-Cell Proliferation," *Yale Journal of Biological Medicine* 55 (1982):437–42.
9. Robert L. Gross and Paul M. Newberne, "Role of Nutrition in Immunologic Function," *Physiological Reviews* 60 (January 1980):188–89, 288–90.
10. R. K. Chandra and P. M. Newberne, *Nutrition, Immunity, and Infection: Mechanics of Interactions* (New York: Plenum Press, 1977), p. 187.
11. W. R. Beisel et al., "Single Nutrient Effects on Immunologic Functions," *Journal of the American Medical Association* 245 (1981):53.
12. *Ibid.*

13. G. H. Bourne, "Vitamin C and Immunity," *British Journal of Nutrition* 2 (1949):341–46.
14. Kenneth H. Falchuk, "The Role of Zinc in the Biochemistry of the *Euglena Gracilis* Cell Cycle," in *Trace Metals in Health and Disease*, ed. Norman Kharasch (New York: Raven Press, 1978), pp. 177–88.
15. Stephen Levine, "Oxidants, AntiOxidants and Chemical Hypersensitivities," part 2. *International Journal of Biosocial Research* 4 (1983):102–5.
16. Beisel, *op. cit.*
17. David S. Rowe, Foreword in Chandra and Newberne, *op. cit.*
18. Donald Rudin, lecture, Orthomolecular Society, Huxley Institute, New York, December 1982.
19. M. G. Brush, "Efamol in the Treatment of the Premenstrual Syndrome," Special Report, Dept. of Gynecology, St. Thomas's Hospital Medical School, London, S.E.1, 1981.
20. Jeffrey Bland, Metabolic Update, Bellevue–Redmont Clinic, Bellvue, WA, July, 1983.
21. Horrobin, *op cit.*
22. William R. Borrmann, *Comprehensive Guide to Nutrition*, second edition (Chicago: New Horizons Publishing Corp., 1979), p. 1.
23. Roy J. Shephard, *Physiology and Biochemistry of Exercise* (New York: Praeger Publishers, 1982), pp. 209–10.
24. Z. Fejfa, "Interrelationships Between Nutrition, Physical Activity, and Cardiovascular Health," in *Nutrition, Physical Fitness and Health*, eds. Jana Parizkova and V. A. Rogoskin (Baltimore: University Park Press, 1978), p. 277.

INDEX

Acetylcholine,
  and relaxation, 163
  and sources, 170
Acid foods, list of, 54
Acne, *see also* Skin, 48–55
  and acid foods, 54
  and avocados, 51
  and cholesterol, 54
  and cortisone, 49
  and dairy products, 50
  and Dilantin, 49
  and essential fatty acids, 51
  and Eugalan Forte, 51
  and exercise, 54
  and fiber, 52
  and gamma linolenic acid, 51
  and hormones, 49
  and ice cream, 49–50
  and intestinal bacteria, 50
  and iodides, 49
  and lactobacillus acidophilus, 51
  and lactobacillus bulgaricus, 50
  and lactobacillus bifidus, 51
  and penicillin, 50
  and processed foods, 54
  and progesterone, 53
  and retinoids, 54
  and sulfur, 53
  and supplements, 53
  and vitamin A, 52
Adams, Ruth, *Did You Ever See a Fat Squir-rel?*, 102

Addictive foods, 76–77
Adipose tissue, *see also* Fat cells, in seden-tary people, 88
Adrenalin, and stress, 74, 163
Aerobics
  definition of, 9
  advantages of, 10–11
Alcohol
  and addiction, 77
  and heart diseasse, 114–15
Allergy
  and dark circles under eyes, 34
  and stress, 166
Aloe vera, 41–43
  as anesthetic, 61
  as toothache remedy, 70
Alopecia, 45–47
  and androgens, 46
  and biotin as cure, 45
  and eggs, 45–46
  and sebaceous glands, 45
  and zinc, 45
Amino acids, *see also* Protein, and mood changes, 206
Analgesics, and nutrient interactions, 209
Androgens, and alopecia, 46
Anemia, 81
Antacids, and nutrient interactions, 209
Antibiotics, and nutrient interactions, 208–9
Anticancer, substances in beta-carotene, 126

Anticancer, substances (*continued*)
  in broccoli, 125
  in vitamin A, 126
  in vitamin C, 126
Anticoagulants, and nutrient
    interactions, 209
Anticonvulsants, and nutrient interactions,
    209
Antidepressants, and nutrient interactions,
    210
Antioxidants
  BHT, 116–21
  B$_{15}$, 118
  vitamin C, 118
  vitamin E, 118
Arthritis
  and B$_6$, 128
  and vegetarianism, 109
Artificial sweeteners, and set point, 96
Ascorbic acid
  and acne, 53
  as antioxidant, 118
  and BHT, 120
  and cancer protection, 126
  and cholesterol, 127
  and drug interactions, 31–32, 208
  and foods, 171
  and free radicals, 127
  and iron absorption, 15–16
  in lettuce, 97
  and menstruation, 192
  and mitochondria, 127
  and wound repair, 61
  and salicylates, 30–31
  and stress, 170
Ascorbic acid, deficiency
  and immunity, 201
  and periodontal disease, 33, 68
  and PMS (premenstrual syndrome), 192
Aspirin, and heart disease, 114–15
Atkins, Robert, *Dr. Atkins Diet Revolution*,
    102
Atopic eczema, and GLA (gamma linolenic
    acid), 55
Autonomic nervous system, and stress, 160
Avedon, Luciana, *The Beautiful People's Diet
    Book*, 103
Avocados, and acne, 51–52

Bacteria, friendly
  lactobacillus acidophilus, 51

lactobacillus bulgaricus, 50
lactobacillus bifidus, 51
Ballentine, M.D., Rudolph, on margarine,
    110–13
Banting, William, *Banting's Diet*, 100
Beans, 130–32
B-cells, and immunity, 198
Benowicz, Robert J., on nutrient-drug inter-
    actions, 207–10
Beta-carotene
  as anti-cancer agent, 126
  and suggested quantity, 205
Bezoza, M.D., Howard, on pre-op care, 60–
    62
BHA, 119
BHT, 116–21
  and ascorbic acid, 120
  and cholesterol, 120
  and the GRAS list, 118
  as supplement, 205
  and vitamin C, 120
Biotin, and hair loss, 45
Bland, Ph.D., Jeffrey
  on aerobic exercise, 9–10
  on margarine, 110–13
  on misleading studies, 36
Body odor, and nutrient remedies, 58
Bone loss, and exercise, 3
Books, on pregnancy and parenting, 215–
    16
Bran, and overutilization, 205
Bread, 133
  and satiety, 123
Broccoli, and cancer, 125
Butter, 112–13
B vitamins
  and carbohydrate metabolism, 17
  in desiccated liver, 33
  and Dilantin interaction, 30
  and fast foods, 139
  and formula guidelines, 204
  and relief of headaches, 62
  and mitochondria, 89
  and potassium metabisulphite, 135
  and weight gain, 89
B vitamins, deficiency causing
  alopecia, 46
  dandruff, 62, 63
  menstruation difficulties, 192
  pellagra, 81
  periodontal disease, 68
  swelling and redness of lips, 33

Caffeine
  and addiction, 77
  and breast lumps, 58
  curtailment for pre-op care, 60–61
  and magnesium interaction, 172
Calcium
  assimilation from milk, 95
  in foods, 145, 194
  and relief of headaches, 62
  and periodontal disease, 68
  and phosphorus ratio, 68
  and suggested quantity, 207
Cancer
  and chemotherapy, 210
  and stress, 166
Capsicum, as toothache remedy, 70
Carbohydrate craving, 89
Cardiopulmonary resuscitation, 39
Carrots, as constipation aid, 149
Cayenne pepper
  as digestive aid, 43
  and menopause, 194
  for sore throat, 43
Chemotherapy, and nutrient interactions, 210
Chick peas, 124
Chocolate, and headaches, 157
Cholesterol
  and acne, 54
  and BHT, 120
  and effect of dairy products, 112
  and GLA (gamma linolenic acid), 211
  and hydrogenated fats, 112
  and immunity, 202
  and stress, 166
  and vegetables, 109
  and vitamin C deficiency, 127
Cholesterol, drugs which lower, and nutrient interactions, 209
Choline, 124
Chromium
  suggested quantity, 207
  and stress, 171
Cis-fatty acids, 146
Citrus fruit, 150–51
Coal-tar dyes, hazards, used in hair coloring, 66
Cod-liver oil
  as source of vitamin A, 53
  as Omega-3 oil, 147
Complex carbohydrates, 14
  and advantages in exercise, 14

and sodium/potassium ratios, 15
Conjunctivitis, 33
Consentino, M.D., Joseph, on image projection and plastic surgery, 59–60
Constipation
  and carrots, 149
  and causes, 190
  and remedies, 190
Cookbooks, recommended list, 215
Cooley, Donald G., *The New Way to Eat and Get Slim*, 101
Corsello, M.D., Serafina, on stress, 159–76
Cott, M.D., Allan, on fasting, 86
Cottage cheese, 136
Cravings
  and addictions, 96
  for carbohydrates, 89
Cultured milk, 50–51

Dairy products
  and acne, 50
  and cholesterol, 112
  and menopause, 195
Dancers, and menarche, 49
Dandruff, 62–65
  and B complex, 62, 63
  and calcium, 62
  and hair sprays, 63
  and processed foods, 65
  and sugar, 63
Daylight exposure, benefits, 8
DES (diethylstilbestrol), and meat, 138
Dental caries, 166
Diabetes
  drugs, and nutrient interactions, 209
  and sugar, 154
Diet, optimal, 177–79
Diet books, 99–105
Diethylstilbestrol, *see* DES
Digestion
  and cayenne pepper, 43
  and stress, 163–64, 165
Diuretics, and nutrient interactions, 209
Dolger, Jonathan, *The Expense Account Diet*, 102
Drugs, and nutrient interactions, 30–32, 207–10
Dufty, William, on sugar, 85

Eczema, atopic, and GLA (gamma linolenic acid), 55

Edema
  allergic, 95
  and food sensitivity, 34
EFA (essential fatty acids)
  and cancer, 211
  deficiencies of, and skin, 34, 82
  and fish, 152
  and hydrogenated fats, 112
  and immunity, 211
  and saturated fats, 53–54
  sources of, 212
  and hydrogenated fats, 112
Eggs
  and alopecia, 45–46, 64
  and heart disease, inverse relationship,
    132
  and pre-op care, 61
  and sodium-potassium ratio, 15
  as victim of anticholesterol establishment,
    113
  and zinc, 91
Emotions, and exercise, 9, 10
Endorphins, 165
Estrogen
  and breast lumps, 58
  and hydration, 61
  and liver function, 192
Eugalan Forte, for acne, 51
Exercise
  and acne, 54
  and age, 10–11
  and anorexia, 26
  and B vitamins, 17
  and bone loss, 3
  as cause of amenorrhea, 4
  as cause of anemia, 5
  as cause of bloody urine, 4
  and complex carbohydrates, 14
  and emotions, 9
  and glucose, 13
  and the heart, 9, 10
  and high density lipoproteins,
    54
  and joggers' nipples, 3
  and lactate, 24–25
  and memory, 11
  and mental function, 10
  and sodium, 15
  and treadmills, 7–8, 16
  and vitamin C, 17
  and vitamin E, 17
  and weight loss, 76
Eyton, Audrey, F-Plan Diet, 104

Fast foods, 139
Fasting, 84–86
Fat cells, causes of, 88
Fat, dietary,
  and effects of processing, 145
  in peanut butter, absorption, 123
  and metabolism in exercise, 87
  and oxidation, 136
Fatty acids, 164
Fever, and immunity, 200
Fiber
  as aid for constipation, 190
  recommended amount, 205, 206
  and vegetarianism, 109
Fiber, lack of, and
  acne, 52
  periodontal disease, 69
Fight or flight, and stress, 162
Filmstrips on nutrition, 216
Fish
  and EFA (essential fatty acids), 152
  and fat content, 97
  and high-density lipoproteins, 152
  and omega-3 oils, 152
  and omega-6 oils, 147
  and zinc, 91
Fisher, Ph.D., Helen E., on exercise and
    anthropology, 18
Flatulence, and food sensitivity, 84
Flossing, 69
Fluid retention,
  Mandell, M.D., Marshall, on, 95–96
  and breast tenderness, 192
Flourescent lights, and melanoma, 38
Folacin
  cooking effects on, 109
  and drug interactions, 31–32
  and PMS (premenstrual syndrome), 59
Folk remedies
  and aloe vera, 41–43
  and cayenne pepper, as digestive and sore
    throat aids, 43
  and honey, as bactericide, 41
  and ice cubes, as analgesic, 43
  and lemons, for foot calluses and skin
    beautifier, 43
  and menopause, 194–95
  and oatmeal, as skin protector, 43
  for toothaches, 70
Food dairy, outline for, 188–89
Food sensitivity, 84
Fredericks, Ph.D., Carlton
  on partially hydrogenated fats, 146

on natural tranquilizers, 173
Free radicals, 117–21
  and oils, 137
  and vitamin C, 127
French Vanilla Frostbite, 38

Garlic, and blood pressure, 114
Gingiva, and nutrients, 68
Ginseng, and menopause, 194
GLA (gamma linolenic acid)
  helpful for
    acne, 52, 53
    atopic eczema, 55
    immune response, 211
    menopause, 195
    menstruation, 193
    PMS (premenstrual syndrome), 59
Glucose
  as fuel for glycogen, 13
  as source of energy, 164
Gluten
  sensitivity to, 84
  and wheat-free menus, 180–88
Glycogen
  as carbohydrate storage, 13–14
  and the untrained athlete, 15
Gold, cost, compared with drugs, 42–43
Gout, medications for, and nutrient interactions, 210
Gray hair
  and dyes, 66
  and PABA, 66
  and pantothenic acid, 66
  and zinc, 66
Gum tragacanth, in meat, 138

Hair dyes, 66
Hair loss, in men, *see* Alopecia
Hair loss, in women, 64
Hall, Ph.D., Ross Hume, on *four food groups*, 139
Hamburgers, 138
Hanley, M.D., Daniel, on muscle function, 15
Hauser, Gayelord, *Diet Does It: You Are What You Eat,* 101
Headache, remedy for, 62
Heart disease
  and alcohol, 114–15
  and aspirin, 114–15

and collagen, 165
and eggs, 132
and exercise, 7, 9, 10, 212–13
and overweight, 92
and sugar, 154
Hemoglobinuria, and exercise, 5–6
Hemorrhoids, and aloe vera, 42
Hexachlorophene, and dangers, 30
High-density lipoproteins
  and exercise, 54
  and fish, 152
  and vitamin C, 127
Hippocrates, 213
Honey, as bactericide, 41
Hot dogs
  and filler meat, 137
  and sodium nitrite, 137
Hummus, 122
Hunger disease, and the Warsaw ghetto, 81
Hunter, Beatrice Trum
  on cottage cheese, 136
  on margarine, 110–13
Hydrogenated fats
  in margarine, 111
  dangers of, 146
  and *trans*-fats, 112
Hypertension, and sucrose, 154
Hypoglycemia
  and glucose in exercise, 13
  and hunger, 81
  and sugar, 154
Hypothalamus, and stress, 159–64

Immunity
  and B-cells, 198
  and fever, 200
  and lymph system, 198–99
  and nutrient deficiencies, 200–2
  and stress, 166, 197–213
  and T-cell production, 198
  and thymus, 197
Inflammation, and aloe vera, 42
Intestinal flora, 50
Iron
  absorption of, 15–16, 33
  and menstruation, 192
Jogging, dangers of
  amenorrhea, 4
  anatomy malfunctions, 4
  anemia, 5
  carbon monoxide, 8
  bloody urine, 4

Jogging, dangers of (continued)
  dehydration, 3
  joggers' nipples, 3
  vascular occlusion, 3
  bronchial spasms, 4

Kamen, Michael, on promoting lifelong habits in children, 23
Kryptopyrrole, the vitamin B$_6$, 171
Kulick, Florence, The Hamptoms Health Spa Diet Cookbook, 105

Lactate, and exercise, 24–25
Lactic acid, see Lactate
Lactobacillus acidophilus, and acne, 51
Lactobacillus bulgaricus, and acne, 50
Lactobacillus bifidus, and acne, 51
Lemons
  and foot calluses, 43
  as skin beautifier, 43
Laxatives, and nutrient interactions, 209
Levin, M.D., Warren
  on supplementation, 203–7
Levine, Ph.D., Stephen, on selenium, 202
Lettuce, and vitamins A and C, 97
Liver, 153
Lubowe, M.D., Irwin, on dandruff, 63
Lymph system, 198–99
  and exercise, 199
Lysine, and viral infections, 206

Magazines, recommended list, 215
Magnesium
  and body odor, 58
  and caffeine, 172
  and free fatty acids, 172
  and suggested quantities, 207
  and smoking, 172
  and stress, 166
Malabsorption, and food sensitivities, 84
Male pattern baldness, see Alopecia
Malonaldehyde
  and beef, 212
  and PUFAs, 211
Mandell, M.D., Marshall
  on water retention, 95–96
  It's Not Your Fault You're Fat Diet, 104
March hemoglobinuria, see Hemoglobinuria

Margarine, 110–13
Meat, 125
  beef and malonaldehyde, 212
  and DES, 138
  elimination of, 125–26
  and gum tragacancth, 138
Melanoma
  and fluorescent lights, 38
  and PCBs (polychlorinated biphenyls), 38
Memory, and exercise, 11
Menopause, 194–95
Menstruation, 191–94
  and dancers, 49
  and vitamin A, 82
Methionine, 124
Milk
  and calcium assimilation, 95
  milk-free menus, 180–87
  skimmed, and problems, 94
  and weight gain, 84
Minerals, and supplementation, 207
Mitochondria, 88–89
  and aerobic exercise, 10
  and vitamin C, 127
Mononucleosis, and stress, 166
MSG, 140–42

Natural food, 143–44
Niacin
  and stress, 17
  and tryptophan, 124
  as tranquilizer, 173
Nutrient deficiencies,
  and impact on immunity, 200
  and lack of quality food, 81
  and periodontal disease, 68
Nutrient density, 97
Nutrients
  and drug interactions, 30–32
Nuts, 133

Oatmeal, use as soap, 43
Obesity, see also Weight gain,
  and conversion of PUFAs, 147
  and definition of, 90–91
  and lack of exercise, 86
  and heart disease, 92
  and metabolism, 82
Oils
  EFA (essential fatty acids), 34, 54, 82, 112, 152, 154, 211, 212

GLA (gamma linolenic acid), 52, 53, 55, 59, 193, 195, 211
omega-3 class, 147, 152
omega-6 class, 147
and rancidity, 136
Oliver, M.D., William, on salt, 154–56
Omega-3 oils, see Oils
Omega-6 oils, see Oils
Optimal diet, 177–79
Oranges, 150–51
Organizations, list of, 216
Osteoporosis, 68, 194

PABA
and body odor, 58
and gray hair, 66
suggested quantity, 205
and suntan, 35
Pantothenic acid
in foods, 171
and gray hair, 66
and immunity, 201
lost in processing, 67
and stress, 171, 173
Parasympathetic nervous system, and relaxation, 160
PCBs (polychlorinated biphenyls), and melanoma, 38
Peanut butter, and fat absorption, 123
Periodontal disease, 68–69
Perspiration, and sodium, 15
Petechia, 39
Pfeiffer, M.D., Carl, on hair strength, 64
Phenytoin, and folate levels, 30
Phosphorus
and processed foods, 68
and role in skeletal tissue, 68
Platelet aggregation, and stress, 213
Potassium, in foods, 172
Potassium metabisulphite, dangers of, 135
PMS (premenstrual syndrome), 59, 191–92
Pre-op program, 60–61
Pritikin, Nathan, The Pritikin Permanent Weight-Loss Manual, 104
Processed foods
and dandruff, 64
and menopause, 195
and oxidative reactions, 136
and salt, 172
Prostaglandins
and sleep, 22
and menstruation, 192

Protein
and amino acids, 164
and amino acid manipulation, 206
in liquid form, 86
and periodontal disease, 68
in powdered form, 86
sources of, 126
Psoralen, dangers of, 37
Psoriasis, 37
Putnam, Nina Wilcox, Tomorrow We Diet, 100

Quieting Reflex, The, 174

Race-walking, see Walking, fast
Rancidity
heat-caused, 146
and oils, 136
and PUFAs (polyunsaturated fatty acids), 145
and sesame seeds, 124
and vitamin E, 145
Rebounding, advantages of, 23
Recipes
avocado omelet, 186
broiled fish, 184
buckwheat pancakes, 185
cauliflower pecan salad, 126
chicken salad, 184
crécy glacé, 148
curried rice, 187
curry dressing, 129
easy millet, 183
egg foo yung, 132
egg foo yung with tofu, 187
fish salad, 186
foie de veau smitane, 153
granola, 187
grated carrot, 184
jambon à la crême, 149
lentil soup, 181
liver slivers, 182
marinated cucumbers, 130
marinated mushrooms, 130
mustard-horseradish dressing, 128
Oriental brown rice, 184
poires belle hélène à la caroube, 153
rice almondine, 133
salad, 181
salade des endives et des oranges, 149

Recipes (*continued*)
  salmon trout, 186
  soup, 186
  soy pancakes, 182
  steamed chicken, 183
  steamed vegetables, 182
  string bean mousse, 184
  sunshine carrot salad, 129
  tamale pie, 130
  tarator soup, 183
  tarte des demoiselles tatin, 154
  tofu omelet, 185
  tomates farcies, 151
Retinoids, and acne, 54
Rice
  forms of, and blood glucose, 123
  and nutrient value, 133

Salicylates, and vitamin C, 30–31
Salt, *see also* Sodium
  and FDA regulations, 156
  and the Yanomama Indians, 154–56
Satiety, and bread, 123
Saturated fatty acids, nonessential dietary,
    list of, 54
Scobey, Joan M., *Short Rations: Confessions
    of a Cranky Calorie-Counter,* 103
Selenium
  and immunity, 202
  recommended amount, 205
Selye, M.D., Hans, on disease resistance,
    165
Semistarvation experiments, 80
Serotonin
  as appetite regulator, 89
  and mood, 171
  and weight reduction, 90
Sesame seeds, 124
Set point, 72–79
  and artificial sweeteners, 96
  and food sensitivity, 84
Skin, *see also* Acne
  and EFA (essential fatty acids), 34
  and rashes, 37–38
  and retinoids, 54
  and vitamin A, 34
Skinfolds, and weight loss, 82
Smith, Richard, *The Bronx Diet,* 103
Smoking
  and addiction, 77
  and aging, 59

and jogging, 3
and magnesium, 172
and pre-op care, 60
and teeth stains, 67
and weight gain, 93
and wrinkles, 34
Sodium, *see also* Salt
  and exercise, 15
  and perspiration, 15
  and stress, 172
  and weight, 79
Sodium hypochlorite, and cottage cheese,
    136
Sodium nitrite, and hot dogs, 137
Soft drinks, and phosphorus, 68
Sore throat, and cayenne pepper, 43
Sprouting, how to, 217
Stern, Judith, *How to Stay Slim and Healthy
    on the Fast Food Diet,* 103
Stone, Ph.D., Irwin, on ascorbic acid, 170–
    71
Stress
  and adrenalin, 74, 163
  and allergy, 166
  and ascorbic acid, 170
  and cancer, 166
  and cholesterol, 166
  and chromium, 171
  and dental caries, 166
  and digestion, 163
  and fight or flight reaction, 162
  and hypothalamus gland, 159
  and immunity, 166
  and magnesium, 166
  and mononucleosis, 166
  and oxygen uptake, 22
  and pantothenic acid, 171, 173
  and sodium, 172
  and thyroid gland, 74
  and triglycerides, 166
  testing, 168–69
  and vitamin B_6, 171
  and weight, 83
  and zinc, 171
Stroebel, M.D., Charles, on *The Quieting
    Reflex,* 174
Sucrose, and hypertension, 154
Sugar
  and addiction, 77
  and allergies, 154
  as antimicrobial agent, 41
  and cavities, 69

and dandruff, 63
and menopause, 195
Sulfa, drugs, and nutrient interactions, 209–
10
Sulfur
and acne, 53
and menopause, 194
and pre-op care, 61
Sun, and aging, 59
Sunburn
and aloe vera, 42
and PABA, 35
and vitamin B$_6$, 35
Sunflower seeds, nutrient value, 129
Sunglass Syndrome, 39
Supplementation
and immunity, 203–7
regimen, 204–7
Sympathetic nervous system, and stress, 160

Taller, Herman, *Calories Don't Count*, 101
T-cell production, and immunity, 198
Thixotrophy, 199
Thymus, and immunity, 197
Thyroid
hormones and nutrient interactions, 209
and menopause, 194
and weight reduction, 74
Toothache, remedies, 70
Trace elements
and antioxidants, 118
and fast foods, 139
and mitochondria, 89
Trans-fats, 112, 146
Triglycerides
and fish, lowering effect of, 152
and stress, 166
Tryptophan
and skin and hair health, 124
as serotonin precursor, 171

Vegetables
and cholesterol, 109
and folate, 109
Vegetarianism, 94
on airlines, 108
and amino acids, 109
and arthritis, 109
and diabetes, 109

and fiber, 109
and its popularity, 109
and a stringent regimen, 110
Vitamin A
and acne, 53
and drug interactions, 31
and dry, flaky skin, 34
and cancer protection, 126
and fast foods, 139
and lettuce, 97
and suggested quantities, 205
Vitamin A, deficiencies causing
lowered immunity, 201
menstruation problems, 82
periodontal disease, 68
PMS, 59
skin problems, 34
Vitamin B$_6$
and acne, 53
and arthritis, 128
and body odor, 58
and drug interactions, 31
and effect of heat, 127
and hair strength, 64
and immunity, 201
and kryptopyrrole, 171
and menstruation, 192
and menopause, 194
and MSG, remedy, 141
and PMS, 59
and stress, 171
and sunburn, 35
and suggested quantities, 204
and sun, 35
Vitamin B$_{12}$
and drug interactions, 31, 32
suggested quantities, 204
Vitamin B$_{15}$, an antioxidant, 118
Vitamin C, *see* Ascorbic Acid
Vitamin D
and skin absorption of, 35
and drug interactions, 31
and periodontal disease, 68
Vitamin E
and acne, 53
as antioxidant, 118
and endurance, 17
and immunity, 201
and menopause, 194
and pre-op care, 61
and rancidity, 145
and stress, 173

Vitamin E (*continued*)
  suggested quantities, 205
  as toothache remedy, 70
Vitamin K
  and drug interactions, 31–32
  and vegetable content of, 125

Walking, fast
  and its advantages, 3–8, 12
  and pre-op care, 61
Warsaw ghetto, 80–82
Water, and pre-op care, 61
Weight gain, *see also* Obesity, 72–79
  and bag of tricks, 92
  and B-complex vitamins, 89
  and milk, 84
  and smoking, 93
  and wheat sensitivity, 84
Weight reduction
  and exercise, 76, 78–79, 87
  and liquid protein, 86
  and powdered protein, 86
  and semistarvation experiments, 80
  and serotonin, 90
  and set point, 72–79
  and skinfold, 82
  and sodium, 79
  and stress, 83

and thyroid, 74
and wheat, 84
and zinc, 91
Williams, Roger, on the synergism of nutrients, 35
Wine, and migraines, 157
Withdrawal symptoms, 77, 84
Whole foods, 122
  and hair loss, 64
  and biological advantages, 122–23

Yanomama Indians, and salt, 155–56
Yellowlees, M.D., Walter, on refined foods, 106–8
Yudkin, M.D., John, on dandruff, 63

Zell oxygen, as source of B complex, 193
Zinc
  and alopecia, 45, 46
  and body odor, 58
  and hair, 64, 66
  and immunity, 201
  and menstruation, 192
  and pre-op care, 61
  and recommended amount, 207
  and stress, 171
  and weight loss, 91